"I recommend this book."

—*Bernie Siegel, M.D.*

"As a medical social worker, I have found *Surviving Cancer* to be full of hope and inspiration for people who have been thrown into the ocean of 'cancer' and are trying to learn how to swim, frequently all on their own."

—*Diane Gorsky*

"A practical, jargon-free guide for anyone facing serious illness, *Surviving Cancer* should be required reading for patients and their doctors!!"

—*Rosanne Shapiro, LICSW*

"In a time when more Americans are questioning the traditional ways of 'Western medicine' and seeking alternative approaches toward healing, Ms. Levine's book could not be more timely and appropriate. This book illustrates beautifully how by incorporating many different styles and techniques, a state of well-being can be obtained."

—*Renee Jacobs, M.D., Ph.D., Internal Medicine,*
Newton Wellesley Hospital and Deaconess Glover Hospital

"As a physician dealing with my own cancer, I am now presented with a new and different challenge. We use your book

in our hospital support group and have found it incredibly helpful. Your spirit of courage, love, and imagination in the face of the dreaded disease helps us touch and catalyze that spirit within each of us. With your excellent suggestions and deep insight we realize we are not alone and can find meaning in the struggle."

—*Dr. Charles Boren, M.D., Department of Psychiatry,*
Former Chief and Medical Director of the Institute for Living,
Hartford, Connecticut

"The range of topics covered is remarkable. From concrete advice about dealing with doctors (e.g., bring someone with you; take a tape recorder), to suggestions for better nutrition, to connecting with nature . . . a unique and superb addition to the literature on wellness."

—*Esther Blank Greif, Ph.D., Psychologist*

Advance Praise for *Surviving Cancer* by Margie Levine

"Margie Levine has written an owner's manual for cancer patients. Her lessons are from the heart and provide a blueprint to overcoming disease. *Surviving Cancer* teaches us how to mature and evolve as we overcome physical and emotional obstacles."

—*Mehmet Oz, M.D., New York–Presbyterian Hospital, author of* Healing from the Heart

"This is a remarkable book—one that reveals the impact of cancer on an extraordinary person who summons the will to survive."

—*David G. Nathan, M.D., President Emeritus, Dana-Farber Cancer Institute, and Robert Stranahan Distinguished Professor of Pediatrics and Professor of Medicine at Harvard Medical School*

"Margie Levine is a woman of courage, a pioneer, and a person saving many lives."

—*David John Sugarbaker, M.D., Chief of Thoracic Surgery, Brigham and Women's Hospital, Professor of Medicine, Harvard University*

"The most remarkable blend of raw useful information coupled to deep inspiration and wonder."

"This is a book for all patients who have chronic or recurring illnesses (arthritis, heart conditions, asthma), or acute problems that are resistant to healing. For physicians, my advice is, give this book to your patients. For patients, give this book to your friends. Take control of your recovery."

"*Surviving Cancer* pays tribute to the real heroes of cancer research. Patients who choose to become involved in investigational research have special qualities that have not been recognized. They show extraordinary courage, determination, and good will in the face of adversity. Margie Levine is a remarkable example. Their absolutely essential, indeed critical contribution to progress in cancer treatment, as is the case for Margie Levine, has not been appreciated and deserves to be told. All effective and curative treatments for cancer that exist today were made possible by such volunteers."

SURVIVING

CANCER

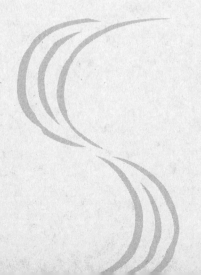

One woman's story and
her inspiring program
for anyone facing a
cancer diagnosis

BROADWAY BOOKS NEW YORK

SURVIVING
CANCER

Margie Levine

BROADWAY

An earlier version of this book was previously published
under the title *Embracing Challenge*.

Broadway Books titles may be purchased for business or promotional use or
for special sales. For information, please write to: Special Markets Department, Random House, Inc., 1540 Broadway, New York, NY 10036.

BROADWAY BOOKS and its logo, a letter B bisected on the diagonal, are
trademarks of Broadway Books, a division of Random House, Inc.

Permissions on p. 236

Visit our website at www.broadwaybooks.com

Designed by Dana Leigh Treglia

Library of Congress Cataloging-in-Publication Data
Levine, Margie, 1946–
Surviving cancer: one woman's story and her inspiring program for anyone
facing a cancer diagnosis / Margie Levine.—1st ed.
p.   cm.
Includes bibliographical references.
1. Levine, Margie, 1957–   —Health.   2. Lungs—Cancer—Patients—
United States—Biography.   3. Mesothelioma—Patients—United
States—Biography.   4. Cancer—Alternative treatment.   I. Title.
RC280.L8 L485 2001
362.1'9699424'0092—dc21
[B]   2001025165

ISBN 0-7679-0715-9

7   9   10   8   6

For Celia

1911–1992

When you have come to the edge
of all the light you know
and are about to step out
into the darkness of the unknown
Faith is knowing that one of two things will happen
There will be something solid to stand on . . . or
You will be taught to fly.

—ANONYMOUS

There is no limit to your being
Only those you ascribe to yourself
There is no limit to your understanding
Only those that are due to trying to understand
with the mind
There is no limit to your light
Except the dark shadows of the ego cast upon the sky
Which we call the self
Shake your soul. Awaken it from slumber.
The time has come to awaken to your divine being.

—PIR VILAYAT INAYAT KAHN

Foreword

"You have cancer."

These are the three most dreaded words a patient can hear from his physician. When faced with the diagnosis of cancer, some patients will experience a wide range of emotions: fear, panic, loneliness, anger, desperation, to name a few. Even when the prognosis is good and treatments are likely to be effective, these reactions occur.

Margie Levine was faced with these words and for her the prognosis was poor. For others with her disease, even aggressive treatments had been ineffective. Still, she endured them. More than that; she literally embraced them—the treatments, her caregivers, and the challenge of fighting her disease. In so doing, she has written the book on *Surviving Cancer,* literally and figuratively.

Margie did not disdain conventional medicine in the hope of a miracle cure. She herself became that miracle through her total involvement and participation in all aspects of her care. She was fortunate in having loving family and supportive friends, but Margie truly took charge of those parts of her recovery that doctors are not always so good at reaching—the soul, the mind, the heart.

Not all cancer sufferers will be fortunate enough to survive their disease, in spite of progress in treatment and continued research. But none will fail to benefit from this book. Anyone with a loved one, a close friend, or a colleague with cancer will be enriched by *Surviving Cancer*. It is a companion, complete with references, resources, practical suggestions, and inspirational wisdom—a guide, a "hand to hold" to confront the most frightening of challenges. No one should have to face this disease alone, and with this book no one will need to.

—KAREN J. MARCUS, M.D.,
ASSISTANT PROFESSOR OF RADIATION ONCOLOGY,
HARVARD MEDICAL SCHOOL

Acknowledgments

This book began twelve years ago in the backseat of our '88 Pontiac. Driving home from New York after meeting with surgeons at Sloan-Kettering, we stopped for coffee. At the convenience store I purchased a purple-lined notebook and pen. I knew then I needed to tell my story, even before it had unfolded. I wrote and cried all the way home. And with years of sheer determination, and the continued blessing of health, my book has finally come to be.

I am grateful to Dr. David Nathan, president emeritus of the Dana-Farber Cancer Institute, who encouraged me to call his agent. My thanks to Jill Kneerim, who became my agent and believed in me, and to my great editor, Jennifer Josephy, at Broadway Books.

A special tribute to Susan Leon, whose enthusiasm, talent, and skill helped see this book to completion.

Thank you for your patience and sensitivity throughout the project. You were wonderful.

I am deeply grateful to my surgeon, Dr. David Sugarbaker, whose shared glimmer of hope and gifted hands helped save my life. He never left my hospital room without a double thumbs-up sign. I thank Dr. Karen Marcus not only for her meaningful addition to the book, but for how she always went out of her way to phone me when I returned home from the hospital after each lung scan to report the findings. Bless you. You were my comforting angel. Thanks as well to Lisa, the radiology coordinator who always found an open slot for me when I needed a new scan. And to Carol, at the Dana-Farber blood desk, whose warmth and candy bowls helped me through. I also want to thank all of the extraordinary doctors, oncologists, nurses, social workers, technicians, and entire medical staff at Brigham and Women's Hospital and the Dana-Farber Cancer Institute for their support.

I owe the greatest thanks to my husband, Ralph, for his profound caring and unconditional love, even when I was at my worst, for the vases of fresh garden flowers by my bedside, the meals he cooked, and for his help in making the self-published version of this book a reality.

My abiding appreciation to all of my family for their soul support, and to my stepsons, Randy, Dan, and daughter-in-law Karin. Your help made a difference. I send Johanne Tragakis blessings for the boundless giving throughout her own illness. I miss you. My heartfelt gratitude to my dear friends, who stood by me, drove me to medical appointments, to nearby beaches, left casseroles on my doorsteps, and were there for me in so many ways; you know who you are. I deeply thank you.

And to the early readers of my book, Jennifer Jordan for her help in thinking out my story, and to those who offered suggestions: Roz Katz, Irene Sperling, Christina Brodie, Susie O'Brien, Joan Pruchansky, Margie Stein, Elaine Kantrowitz, Linda Clary, Marvin Pave, Beth Bosman, Pearl Lampert, Anne Agnew, Robyne Kurland, Marylou Tschirch, Monique Martel, Judy Taub, Joanne Chmielinski, Carolyn Young, Jan Silverman, and Ginny Reiser. I thank you.

Finally, I want to thank my parents, Joseph Plotka, whose life was taken by cancer and who never lived to see me grow up; your spirit is with me. And to my late mother Celia, a role model of tenacity and creativity, who inspired me to write my story. Her lifelong goal was to one day publish *her* book. *This is for you, Mom.*

Contents

Introduction

Illness is private territory. There is in some who have survived "the worst" an almost transcendent freedom, while in others there is a lingering trauma that drives them into silence, underground. That is because despite your return to health—the clean CAT scans, the normal bloodwork, the clear X rays—the memory of having known hell's inner circle remains. "That is the fearful part of having been near death," wrote Katherine Mansfield. "One knows how easy it is to die. The barriers that are up for everybody else are down for you. You've only to slip through."

For nine years the no-man's land that Mansfield describes governed my life, for although against all expectations I had survived mesothelioma, the rarest and most aggressive form of lung cancer, I rarely spoke of it. Only close friends and family knew about my ordeal. Still traumatized from the experience, I kept it as my secret.

Then in June 1998 I received a phone call from the Dana-Farber Cancer Institute asking me to speak at their gala Society Dinner. I would be sharing my story with hundreds of people, including no fewer than 150 Boston physicians, a Nobel Prize winner in medicine, and several dozen corporate presidents. I was honored yet nervous, for it was the first time I would be openly discussing my battle with cancer. Yet, I knew I had to go, that it was right for me to break that long silence.

The same evening after the phone call I sat in my favorite armchair with pen and paper in hand to begin organizing my thoughts. I spotted a book on a nearby table I'd been wanting to read. As I opened to the first page, I was struck by a quote from the famous mythologist Joseph Campbell, which read: "We must be willing to get rid of the life we have planned, so as to have the life that is waiting for us."

These words resonated instantly with my being. I stopped for a moment. I reflected on my life and realized that, yes, for a while, I had lived the full and rewarding life I had planned.

I had completed graduate school and become a health education coordinator and social worker in the public schools. I taught college psychology classes and ran parent education seminars on the side. I played tournament-level tennis and ran six miles a day. I designed greeting cards for upscale boutiques and vacationed in exotic places. Then I had gotten married, and was planning to start a family.

What I was unprepared for was the life that was waiting for me. That life began at midnight in late October 1989. I was lying in a hospital bed at Massachusetts General Hospital and remember when the surgeon entered my room. Still dressed in bloodstained scrubs, it was evident I was his last call for the night and he was preparing to go home. As he spoke to me he struggled to balance his jacket and bulging briefcase between my bed rail and his hip.

"Your X rays show that large grapefruit tumor on your left lung is asbestos cancer or mesothelioma," he said calmly. "It is a deadly cancer. Unfortunately, we have no cure. We can only palliate."

My head sank back into my pillow as I tried to stifle my sudden urge to gag.

"Surgery is brutal and the recovery long and painful. You may want to forgo treatment and live out your remaining months with dignity and quality of life. Only you can make the decision."

The surgeon answered a few questions, such as what physical changes I could expect in the short time left to me, before cradling his briefcase under his arm and making his escape. Lying there, I was overcome with raw terror as my mind tried to comprehend how dramatically fate had turned my life around in a matter of days.

Then I remembered my elderly mother—blind, but feisty and independent—asleep one floor below. Just weeks before, she had required emergency surgery to remove a kidney. My husband Ralph and I had brought her here to Boston for the best medical care in the country and to be close to her support system, her only child: me.

A long few weeks it had been. As Ralph and I scrambled to be with her and to find her postoperative care at home, I had brushed aside the signs reminding me I wasn't feeling well either. I was more tired than usual and was experiencing shortness of breath and sudden pain in my chest. One day on my way to see Mom I felt a sharp piercing pain near my heart. Not having a cardiologist, I quickly rummaged through the yellow pages and called a doctor who could see me that afternoon. He diagnosed a stress-related inflammation of the muscle around the heart and gave me pills for the pain. "Relax," he said, as he handed me the prescription. It was a road I had been down before.

When I was thirty-two, three disks in my lower back suddenly and irrevocably gave out. I learned how to readjust my life to accommodate the incapacitation and pain. Then, a decade later, my left hand started to tingle and tremble, and I was dizzy. I knew something was not right, yet tests showed nothing. Later, I realized the tingling was from the lung tumor pressing on my spine, but at the time the doctor treating me concluded, "Ma'am, there's not a thing wrong with you. Get over your back problems and get a life," as if my suburban life was so dull I had invented a set of phantom symptoms for company. Insulted, infuriated, and scared, I looked that cold man in the eyes and said, "Doctor, you are wrong."

Two years later, intuitively I knew this diagnosis was

wrong, too. Determined to find out what the piercing pains were, I asked my mother's physician if he could arrange a chest X ray.

"A large mass on the left lung," he stated a few hours later. I was admitted to that hospital the following day for tests and a biopsy to determine where this tumor had originated and if it had spread.

Over the next two weeks, I was poked, prodded, and scanned. Each night I was wheeled down to visit my brave mother, my hospital pajamas concealed under a buttoned trench coat so she couldn't feel them as we embraced each other in a hug. She marveled at the swarms of visitors she received, mostly my friends who traveled between our rooms. Yet she never discovered that I was an inpatient there, or what was really going on. My only goal was to protect her from the anguish and allow her body time to heal. If my news was bad, I prayed that God would give me time to just outlive her.

But malignant pleural mesothelioma, I would learn, does not wait. Not widely recognized until the 1960s, it remains a killer today. This asbestos-related carcinoma grows with weedlike speed and strength through and around the mesothelial tissues of the chest cavity. Ten years ago surgeons facing this disease thrashed about searching for an effective protocol that would halt the spread of this cancer. Even now, most are still reluctant even to attempt an operation.

A casual look at the medical literature I read just after my diagnosis suggests why: "Death usually occurs four to twelve months after diagnosis. . . . Standard management approaches have provided limited effectiveness. . . . Only a small percentage of patients are eligible for surgery; of those 15 percent survive five years with a median survival of sixteen months. . . . Commonly fatal . . . Mortality remains high . . . Poor survival . . . To date, no standard treatment exists. . . ." In other words, the massive asbestos tumor would continue to grow and within months take over my body.

As I lay in my hospital bed late that October night, trembling in the wake of the surgeon's pronouncement, I remember reaching for a Hershey's Kiss from a growing stack of chocolate boxes on my nightstand and thinking, I can enjoy this now, without guilt. I felt my cheeks pucker as I savored the satisfying instant. For a moment I felt free.

Then suddenly the moment of pleasure faded and I had to confront the truth: I was forty-three and I was dying. I knew I needed to get my affairs in order. Days later I began to write farewell letters, phone old acquaintances, say good-bye to dear friends. I hired a lawyer to prepare my will. I discarded secret diaries, gave away a treasured antique doll, my music collection, and my grandmother's pendant watch. But I never gave up hope.

Instead of preparing for death, I started that very night from my hospital room battling to live, calling everyone I knew, networking. I continued between yet more tests, scans, and blood work, to call my friends and their friends, to learn about my disease, find its specialists, and discover my options. I called medical centers, alternative clinics, cancer hotlines, and clergy. At home, there were more conversations, often going late into the night. I decided I would get three opinions. Finally, I found an aggressive mesothelioma treatment and surgeon at New York's Memorial Sloan-Kettering Cancer Center who agreed to operate on me.

But she was in New York, and I knew in my heart that being close to my friends and family in Boston would be essential to my care. Fortunately, with persistence, I was able to convince Dr. David Sugarbaker, a well-known thoracic surgeon at Brigham and Women's Hospital, to perform a variation of the harsh procedure. Dr. Sugarbaker specialized in my type of cancer and was one of the three doctors I had gone to see. But his protocol was pneumonectomy (removing the entire lung), and for some reason, this treatment had not felt right to me. When I asked Dr. Sugarbaker if he would consider the New York protocol, he implied I might not have much of a chance. But I persisted in my requests, and finally he agreed. "Let us get you two years," Dr. Sugarbaker told me, "and maybe by then we'll have found a cure." I held on to that hope like a lifeline. Two years sounded now like an eternity.

The radical treatment lived up to its rigorous billing, and then some. My surgery began with an eighteen-inch incision from my upper spine around to my breastbone. My skin was then folded back and clamped into place with stainless steel clothespins. Next, my bottom two ribs were cracked and removed, opening the entire chest cavity. Now, the surgeon, oncologist, pulmonologist, cardiologist, pathologist, and the day's assortment of residents peered into the hole, searching for any metastasis.

Once convinced the surgery was "worth it," they went

to work. Wielding their scalpels carefully, they removed the tumor and a thick slice of the surrounding tissue to get as much of the vinelike cancer as possible. Then, they peeled the pleura—the lung lining—off the diseased lung and off the remaining healthy organ as well. The pericardium—the sac surrounding the heart—was also separated from the heart while affected portions of the diaphragm were removed. Next, a synthetic chest wall made of mesh was built, fastened together by a hundred or more metal clips. Finally, before they closed me up, they poured as much lethal chemotherapy into the cavity as they dared without killing me on the table. The deadly toxin seeps into all the crevices in the chest cavity, like heat-seeking missiles finding elusive cancer cells the eye cannot.

A fair number of patients do not survive this operation. Because I did, it inspired me to take further action. What I did next forms the core of this book.

My past experiences as a teacher and social worker gave me a base to begin to pull a creative program together. I used my own ideas, my training, my schooling, my reading, and my instincts. I tried to draw on everything and anything I had known that could help guide me. Ironically, the back injury that had brought my active life to a halt for nearly two years, would be my most important teacher. It taught me how to improvise. I learned to take ambulances to hospitals when I couldn't move. I learned how to keep a cooler under my bed with sandwiches and juices so I didn't have to get up. I worked the phone and organized my friends for potluck suppers at my house, so I wouldn't have to cook. I made sure I would be in touch with the outside world and have companionship, so I could remain optimistic and hopeful.

Through crisis we can grow. We can learn to look inside ourselves, to find pieces of our past, to tap our inner wisdom to soften the journey ahead. By embracing the mystery we open ourselves to the diverse ways of healing around us.

Told I was going to die, I never stopped fighting. I never stopped persisting and striving to free myself of this disease and to live every available moment with gusto— whether those moments could be measured by the handful or across a lifetime. Today, two exploratory surgeries, one major operation, five inpatient rounds of chemotherapy, twenty-five radiation sessions, and forty-one healing steps later, I am the world's longest-living survivor of mesothelioma lung cancer. As word of my success with the program that helped bring me back from the precipice spread among Boston-area oncologists, surgeons, patient communities, and then worldwide, I began to receive phone calls from the newly diagnosed. *How did you do it?* they would ask, and I would tell them.

I described how I decided to become my own advocate and how I worked hard integrating traditional medicine with complementary techniques; how I created a personal visualization tape, made an affirmation journal, learned to meditate, and envisioned cancer cells leaving my body through my pores.

I told them about the acupuncture, the energy healer, the hypnotist, the prayer hotlines, and all those glorious picnics by the sea. I spoke of how I coped during those endless hours lying in stuffy MRI tunnels, mentally turning the loud banging into scenes of floating angels hammering away at my tumor with golden axes. I explained how I envisioned the cancerous mass shrinking cell by cell and how I used my mind continually to take charge.

And I described how spiritually connected I became, suddenly seeing the world with new eyes. I had every expectation of dying. Instead, after twelve miraculous years, I am alive and well, living each day with boundless gratitude.

Soon, the calls became more than I could handle. So I put my "Forty-one Steps to Wellness" into a manual I self-published called *Embracing Challenge*. It was a real kitchen-table operation, as the requests came in faster than I could staple the pages together. Friends came over to help take phone calls and stamp and address envelopes. Patients called with questions and told their stories. I was asked to speak at local hospitals, to nurses' associations, on television, on radio. Hospitals in Boston, and beyond, began ordering my manual by the case to give to their cancer patients. And I started working with physicians at several area hospitals, training them in the use of my integrative medicine steps. Last month a surgeon in the audience came running up to me in his blue scrubs after I had finished my presentation, his surgical mask still dangling from his neck. He kissed me on the cheek and said, "You were awesome! I need to go back to the operating table."

Most nights I am up past midnight sending copies of my manual—which I have enriched and expanded here—

around the globe. With this new book, I continue the work of reorienting my life to be a source of hope for many more thousands of cancer patients.

"I dwell in possibility," the poet Emily Dickinson told us. I do, too. With the help of the following chapters, with their simple, life-affirming tools, may you, too, find your way toward healing. I wish for you the balance of action and purpose to displace despair, the inspiration to activate your unique inner strengths, and the motivation to take charge.

Nature takes good care of us, by and large, but we must also take care of ourselves. We must look for the first ray of light, as night gives way, and then another, and another. As you embark on your journey, may each of these pages be a beacon of light. And may you discover your own path to inner peace.

1

Network, Network,

Network!

When facing a major health crisis, connecting with people is an invaluable lifeline. The first weeks after learning you have cancer can feel as if you've been spun around in a whirlwind. You have a diagnosis, and the newness of what's ahead of you may seem overwhelming. Yet decisions need to be made: which physician, which hospital, which protocol, which postoperative treatment plan. No matter how much you've accomplished in your life, now you have to begin again. You have to ground yourself and become educated, perceptive, and receptive. One of the best ways to do that is by networking.

When I was first diagnosed with a rare form of cancer I was unprepared as to how to begin the fight for my life. Instinctively I began calling friends in the medical field, and then friends of *their* friends.

I contacted hospitals, libraries, and cancer clinics. I phoned cancer organizations and holistic health centers. I reached out to people who had been there. I communicated nonstop from my hospital bed phone.

Asking a lot of questions and listening carefully was my strongest tool for survival in those early days. The aggressive nature of my disease meant I needed to take immediate action. Through networking, I found contacts who helped find the appropriate institutions, the best doctors, and a fitting protocol—the contacts that saved my life.

When you are networking you are reaching out for help. You are reaching out for opinions and searching for information that often may be more immediately useful to you than what you can find in books, because it is first-hand, people-driven, up-to-date, and customized to your specific situation by the questions you ask. Very often you can find out a lot of things that might not be easily said or learned in any way other than by shared experience. Cancer makes "fellow travelers" of the people it touches. By seeking out others, we shorten the learning curve. I benefited enormously from the time people took to speak with me, from their advice, honesty, and encouraging words.

I found that connecting with people who have had a

similar type of illness was especially helpful. I also called medical centers and asked if they were familiar with my particular illness, and if they knew any good doctors who specialized in this area. I learned to ask specific questions, evaluate the responses, and to then decide what would work best for me.

For instance, when speaking with other patients, as I tried to get an understanding of what I was facing, I would ask how they had experienced their surgeries and treatments. I asked for their frank opinions about their physicians and how they were treated by them as patients. I wanted to know how receptive a doctor was to new ideas. Did he return phone calls? Rush through consultations and checkups? You may hear excellent things about a physician but have difficulty getting an appointment. I would call doctors I knew to ask if they could help me make a connection that might get me in faster, or ask the nurse practitioner if she had any suggestions. By learning to ask I almost always found important leads that helped open doors.

You will want to inquire about the hospital and how satisfied your networking contacts were with the level of care they received. Did they have any complaints about the staff, about the attention given, about the care and concern that were shown. I asked if they had primary care nursing (where each patient is assigned a head nurse to oversee all of one's care), about the food, parking, and visiting policies. And I asked for any suggestions that might make the anticipated ordeal ahead go more smoothly.

Connecting with others is important because it helps locate many of the pieces that allow for decision-making and creating a plan. I chose three doctors, each at a different medical center, to see for an evaluation. Networking helped mobilize the strength within me so I could begin to move forward.

Working "the Net"

While there is no substitute for the sound of the human voice when confronting challenge, the Internet (nonexistent during this period of my life) offers a gold mine of information on specific cancers, personal experiences, new treatments, and clinical studies.

Many major medical centers, such as the Mayo Clinic and Massachusetts General Hospital, now have their own websites. One particularly good one is OncoLink *(http://oncolink.upenn.edu)*, which is sponsored by the University of Pennsylvania Cancer Center.

Healthfinder *(www.healthfinder.gov)* is a government-sponsored site that is extremely consumer friendly, offering links to hundreds of relevant organizations, centers (such as the National Cancer Institute) and to news services that follow the latest developments in health and medicine. Another government site, MEDLINE *(www.nlm. nih.gov/databases/freemedl/html)*, will summarize new treatments and the evidence collected from specific studies as reported in medical journals, while Alternative Health News Online *(www.altmedicine.com)* and Ask Dr. Weil *(www.drweil.com)* are excellent sources for investigating complementary treatments.

Calling Cancer Fax ([301] 402-5874) will connect you to a computer in Bethesda, Maryland, home of the National Institutes of Health, where you can get information on your particular type of cancer from a fax line. It is chock full of good information.

If you are not comfortable initiating computer searches, ask a friend or family member to look for you, or enlist the help of your local librarian. Try to be as specific as you can when networking on-line. Choosing the appropriate key words can be much like selecting the right bait. The Net is an ocean fathomable though deep. You want to find what's most relevant to your particular circumstances.

In the middle of this road we call our life,
I found myself in a dark wood,
With no clear path through.
—DANTE, *INFERNO*

Since we cannot change reality, let us change
the eyes that see reality.
—NIKOS KAZANTZAKIS,
REPORT TO GRECCO

2

Second and
Third Opinions

There are many approaches to treating disease. By pulling all of your information together and accessing your own intuitive knowledge, you will make the best final choice.

When choosing a hospital it is important to remember that the big cities tend to have the larger hospitals with more well-trained medical specialists and surgeons aboard. In general, those that are teaching hospitals (meaning they are affiliated with medical schools) use more state-of-the-art equipment along with the most advanced techniques. Most important, in larger hospitals there is a stronger likelihood that doctors there have performed your procedure more often than have doctors at smaller hospitals, and with better success rates. Experience is very important when it comes to complicated or unusual cases, but in *any* case, you need to feel confidence in the surgeon you select.

I felt it was important to deal with established institutions and was willing to travel to find the top-notch resources. I sought opinions from three respected medical centers within a six-hour drive from my home. Two were in Boston, Massachusetts General and Brigham and Women's Hospital; and I went to Memorial Sloan-Kettering Cancer Center in New York for my third evaluation. I always checked to make sure the physician I was seeing was board-certified. This means that the doctor has completed both an approved residency program and passed a detailed written exam. The American Board of Medical Specialities ([846] 491-9091 or *www.abms.org*) can provide this information and should be consulted regardless of whether you have managed care insurance and need to select your surgeon from a preapproved list of names, carry free-choice insurance, or have the financial resources to go out-of-network. (Note: Some hospitals provide free care if you have no insurance and limited financial resources. For instance, the Dana-Farber Cancer Institute in Boston will provide services free of charge depending on your income and financial status.)

You may also contact other organizations to learn more about your doctors. The American College of Surgeons ([312] 202-5000 or *www.facs.org*) can tell you if your doctor is a member or fellow of this group (to qualify for membership as a fellow, he or she would have had to pass a peer-review evaluation), while the American Medical Association ([312] 464-5000 or *www.ama-assn.org*) can provide information on your doctor's residency training and medical school education. Your state medical board can tell you whether the doctor you are considering has been the subject of previous disciplinary action.

Sometimes you don't know how many opinions you will want to get before making a decision. I scheduled appointments with several specialists in advance, realizing I could cancel them if they were not necessary. Knowing that the time was being held for me provided a certain sense of security. Having options and a plan of action was comforting. (If you decide to cancel an appointment, be courteous and do so at your earliest opportunity.)

I ordered and personally paid for copies of all my X rays. Many health insurance companies do not cover duplicating costs. I inquired before seeing each new physician as to whether they wanted my films forwarded a week ahead of time. Some doctors appreciate the opportunity for a preliminary patient assessment before the actual consultation. Otherwise, I hand-carried the films to each appointment rather than entrusting the lab or the hospital courier staff to deliver them.

When surgery was suggested I felt comfortable questioning the surgeon as to how many operations of that particular type he had performed. Because my particular form of cancer was rare as well as aggressive, I understood that most doctors see no more than one or two mesothelioma cases in their lifetimes. I wanted to find a thoracic surgeon experienced as well as skilled in cases such as mine. As I spoke with different doctors, I also inquired about the overall success and complication rates from each procedure they offered. It is also important to ask:

- *What are my options?* (We feel better and more in control when we have alternatives, and there usually are.)
- *What are the pros and cons of this procedure?* (Ask this about every option.)
- *How many cases like mine have you seen?*
- *What are the possible consequences if I decide to postpone surgery and wait for a while?*
- *If I were friend or a loved one, what would you advise me to do?* (Most people will ask, What would you do if you were in my situation? a stock question that usually elicits a stock response. The first question almost always prompts a *personal* one.)

As you are likely to be consulting with several physicians during a relatively concentrated period, to avoid confusion try to listen carefully and take diligent notes. Remember to ask similar questions of each doctor you see, so you're not comparing apples and oranges. This way, you will be organized and ready when it's time to make decisions.

It was important to me to gather as much information as I could. It gave me a sense of control and established a mindset that sometimes there are no right answers. This permitted me to be receptive to hearing about new proto-cols. Although not fully tested, some may offer valuable help. In my case, experimentation saved my life.

I also sought information and opinions on how tradi-tional medical and complementary approaches might be brought together creatively. Integrated medicine incorpo-rates the idea that our bodies are more than machines that break down and require repair. Rather, it sees human beings as systems of energy, including emotional as well as spiritual components. It is a point of view gaining wide acceptance in medical circles, a blending of traditional medicine with complementary therapies that enhance the medicine we grew up with. More than sixty medical schools nationwide, including Harvard Medical School and the University of Arizona at Tucson (well known for its affiliation with the physician and author Dr. Andrew Weil), now offer instruction in integrative medicine. When you are in the process of choosing a physician to treat you, ask them their opinions regarding alternative approaches, and how open they are about working with complementary-care practitioners. Do they advocate acu-puncture for help in tolerating chemo treatments? Are they receptive to massage as a way of releasing body toxins? If you choose to supplement your care with complemen-tary therapies, in many instances your doctor's authoriza-tion will be required before your insurance carrier will agree to cover the costs.

When deciding what protocol or combination of treat-ments are going to be right for you, you may find it helpful, as I did, to brainstorm first. I asked a group of my close friends and family to come to my home one evening to help me sift through the information I'd gathered. It has been said that the best way to overcome fear is to make a decision. A close circle of supporters, intimates, or caring friends often adds clarity—and affirmation—to that process.

Locating Alternative Treatment Centers

The list of quality providers of complementary care is growing daily. Contact your local hospital or closest medical center first. More and more institutions have their own hospital-based clinics offering alternative treatments to their patients. The following well-known centers are geographically distributed and may be contacted for a referral near where you live.

- New York. Department of Complementary Medical Services, New York Presbyterian Hospital ([212] 305-9628 or *www.nyp.org*).
- New York. Division of Wellness and Chronic Illness/Division of Family Medicine at University Hospital and

Medical Center, Stonybrook
([631] 444-0624 or
www.uhmc.sunybc.edu/fammed).

- Boston. The Mind-Body Clinic and
  Institute, Beth Israel Deaconess Medical Center ([617] 632-9535 or
  www.mindbody.harvard.edu).
- Cincinnati. The Alliance Institute for
  Integrative Medicine, The Health
  Alliance of Greater Cincinnati
  ([513] 791-5521 or
  www.health-alliance.com).
- Pittsburgh. The Center for Complementary Medicine, University of Pittsburgh Medical Center-Shadyside
  ([412] 623-3023 or fax [412] 623-6414).
- Chicago. Block Medical Center,
  Evanston, Illinois ([847] 492-3040 or
  www.blockmed.com).
- Tucson. The University of Arizona Program in Integrative Medicine
  ([502] 626-7222 or
  www.integrativemedicine.arizona.edu).
- San Francisco. The Institute for Health
  and Healing, California Pacific Medical
  Center ([415] 600-1374 or
  www.cpmc.org).

3

Choose an Advocate

There are a multitude of details that need to be attended to, assessed, and watched over. Even with the most competent of medical teams and in the best of hospitals, it is easy for errors to occur—double-booked appointments, misplaced films, problems with insurance. The paperwork alone can be daunting. For many people, having an advocate involved in the process of making and confirming appointments, organizing test schedules, following up biopsy results, shepherding X rays, overseeing surgery procedures, drug combinations, chemo treatment dates, and home health care aids is a crucial piece of the recovery process.

Having a plan is essential. I am a strong person and like to be in control. Recognizing this made me decide to take charge of my health care. Learning to be vigilant can be an all-consuming job, a matter, literally, of life and death. Illness is a draining experience, but the day-to-day responsibility of overseeing my actual care was one I chose not to delegate. To carry it off I needed to stay very focused. For me, the benefits of actively managing my appointments, test results, medications, and so on made me feel that all my efforts were constructively concentrated on healing. It was how I performed best.

If the role of "mission commander" was not comfortable for me, I would have entrusted someone else to direct my medical care. When looking for an advocate, you are seeking a person who will be part manager, part scheduler. That person needs to be patient, thorough, responsible, steady, confident, organized, have an understanding of your condition and the time and energy to invest in the process. That person may be a partner, a friend, a neighbor, or someone you pay.

During the time I was sick, I was supported from afar by a friend living in the South, who was herself struggling with the same form of cancer. Our regular phone calls and frequent visits were a precious source of emotional nourishment. Her approach to illness was quite different from mine: she made few decisions regarding her day-to-day care. Her husband filled the role of advocate, and he did it quite ably. When we discussed this choice over the phone

one day, she explained it was helpful for her to keep her distance so that she could focus on other aspects of her recovery. She felt it kept her mind clear, her energy up, her emotions cocooned. Our styles differed; she didn't know when her next oncologist visit was scheduled. Yet she felt entirely comfortable. For her, it was an effective game plan.

Each of us develops a different set of survival rules. Whether we heal best keeping our distance from tedious details, or attacking them by taking control, *one person must be fully in charge*. Decide which way will be right for you. Trusting an advocate to do the job can make the ordeal ahead go more smoothly.

4

Medical Notebook

I purchased a small notebook to keep with me at all times. Writing down my thoughts and questions before each doctor visit made me less nervous once I arrived. I kept an ongoing list of questions with me at all times, and whenever I thought of something I wanted to ask about, I'd pull out my notepad and add it to the list. Asking questions helped me to feel more engaged with my treatment and that in turn made me more composed.

Sometimes, as I prepared for an appointment, I wasn't sure what to expect. The stress and the mystery attached to illness and its treatment had an intimidating effect. My mind would literally go blank. So I would begin by asking myself, What are the things I want to know? Invariably, a list of ideas logically followed. I would refine my questions so that when I asked them they were clearly worded and to the point.

I also took notes after each consultation and added them to the notes I had taken in preparation for the visit. That way I had a record of every session—my questions and the doctor's responses. This allowed me to track my progress.

The list of questions I asked included:

- How painful will the surgery/treatment be?
- How long will I be incapacitated?
- When will the anesthesia wear off?
- When will I be able to resume my normal daily activities?
- Will I be able to resume normality in a particular body function, or how (and for how long) will that be compromised?
- Will I go home with pain medicine?
- Will I have to go on a special diet (i.e., to counter constipation)?
- How will the anesthesia affect my bodily functions for the next two weeks after surgery?
- Will the drugs I'm given interfere with the medicine I'm currently taking?
- What side effects can I anticipate?

- Will the side effects/medication interrupt my sleeping pattern and will I need sleeping pills?
- Is there another patient who has been through this surgery and treatment I can speak with?

Your need to be organized extends to the preparations you make as you get ready to enter the hospital, a time when you are understandably distracted and it is easy to forget routine housekeeping concerns. My surgery was followed by extensive chemotherapy that required multiple hospital stays. So I also created additional notebook checklists of necessary tasks or errands I needed to perform prior to or subsequent to my hospital stays. I made a note to change my answering machine message leaving a friend's number if the call was urgent. I wrote down errands to be done: such as bringing foods into the house that I could tolerate during recovery. I jotted down any previously scheduled appointments that needed to be canceled. I listed the items to place on my bedtable for when I returned from the hospital: a water pitcher and paper cups, vitamins and prescription meds, Kleenex, magazines, along with pen and pads by the phone. If you live alone, you may need to ask yourself questions such as: Should I cancel the newspaper? The cleaning lady? Ask a friend to water the plants? Leave a key with a neighbor? Have the post office hold the mail or appoint someone to pick it up and bring it over? Set up timers on my lights? Lower the thermostat?

I made a list of items to pack for overnight hospital stays—my own comfortable robe and slippers, my favorite herbal tea bags, my tape recorder so I could listen to soothing music and to my personal visualization tape, Life Savers, magazines, and writing paper—and kept a bag packed so it would be ready to go next time. And I made a phone list of family, friends, and neighbors to contact from the hospital, as well as a "just in case" list of important phone numbers like those of my next-door neighbor, the building superintendent, the drugstore, and the insurance company—all in deference to this simple truth: you don't want to have to worry about what you may have forgotten. Preparing lists and checklists for your medical notebook reduces your mental clutter and the stress attached to your hospital stay.

Having a list of questions to ask as you prepare to be discharged allows the transition from hospital to home to go smoothly. I always made sure the labeled instructions on the prescription medication bottle I was being sent home with were clear. I would be sure to ask questions if they were not. I would then write the instructions in my notebook in my own words.

I also kept a record of offered treatment options, suggested medications, and follow-up appointment dates. Over time, I added a section where I could add health articles I had clipped to share with my medical team, the names of recommended books to buy, and announcements of dates about patient workshops. And I found a calendar with a "Month at a Glance" feature so that I could always anticipate what was coming. I used my medical notebook continuously, for it made me organized during a most chaotic time.

5

Mini-Tape Recorder

I bought a pocket-size tape recorder to record and recall discussions during appointments with my doctors. Even with diligent note-taking it is difficult to remember and digest the overload of information from any one session. Playing back the conversation afterward in the quiet of my home—sometimes more than once, sometimes replaying the tape for trusted friends and advisers—and knowing I could take the time I needed to assimilate the information, options, and opinions offered was very helpful. It allowed me to respond more rationally, and less emotionally, than I otherwise might have, as doctor's offices were locations where I always experienced a high level of stress.

When you use a tape recorder, consider adding follow-up comments of your own about the session. This can help you to clarify your thoughts. You may also want to use it to make a list of questions for follow-up or for clarification. All consultations and entries of any kind should be dated.

I found tape recorders that come with auto-reverse and earphones the easiest to use. Don't forget to make sure your batteries are fresh!

Note: You must always ask permission before you begin to tape another person. Courtesy and the laws of some states require it. Although many physicians do not like to be recorded, you can alleviate their concerns by explaining you want to avoid confusion about their advice by being able to play it back rather than relying on note-taking. If the doctor remains resistant to your request, it is always important to respect his or her wishes.

6

Bring a Buddy

Having a caring person accompany me to medical appointments offered invaluable support. Trying to ease the burden my husband felt of needing to always be there worked well when I asked trusted friends and family members to come along. If the person was comfortable sitting in during the physical exam, I'd usually invite her to join us.

More important, I'd always ask my companion to sit in with the physician and me during the conversation that followed, whether or not I was tape recording it. It's natural mentally or emotionally to detach when the stakes are high. You can be so tense you don't always hear things correctly. What the doctor is saying may go right over your head; you may hear what you want to hear or block information that is threatening. The comfort of having someone close by your side at a most frightening time offers security and emotional support and helps keep you grounded. Reflecting on the visit afterward with that person can also offer additional clarity. The feedback is useful when making crucial choices and deciding on an appropriate course of action. Even just knowing a friend with a shoulder to lean on is in the waiting room when you come out can make a difference.

7

Self-Empowerment

It was important for me to learn about my specific cancer. Getting information was difficult, for I was an inpatient when initially diagnosed and the doctors and nurses seemed reluctant to provide it. Only in retrospect was I able to understand they were trying to *protect* me from the gruesome data regarding my disease. They didn't understand that I feel more comfortable when I am fully informed and that I have always subscribed to the adage "knowledge is power."

Finally, a friend went to a medical library to obtain further information and I called cancer agencies, which mailed me pamphlets. I read about the experimental drugs and protocols and their predicted side effects. I reviewed the statistics and available research. Becoming familiar with the new medical terminology as well as with the facts about my disease helped me feel empowered. It enabled me to converse more intelligently with the surgeons I met with at the medical centers in New York and Boston, and helped guide me through the all-important decisions I was making as I prepared to battle for my life.

As I evaluated my options, I reviewed the research I had done. I weighed various factors: the procedures offered; the geographic considerations; the surgeons' familiarity with my particular disease; the statistics on success rates given to me. Then I quieted myself and focused on the choices. I listened to how my body spoke to me, the visceral feelings that called out to me as I reviewed the protocols.

After great deliberation I chose to stay in Boston for treatment, for I had a strong support system and wanted to be at home. I was conflicted, however, for when I tuned into my *inner* voice, the surgery being presented to me, which involved removing my lung, did not feel right. Nonetheless, that was the preferred surgical treatment offered in the Brigham and Women's Hospital. I had little choice.

And yet I could not stop thinking about the New York protocol, where mainly the lung lining and tumor were excised, immediately followed by a chemo bath poured directly into the site, followed by radiation at a later date. Somehow I just *knew* that was the treatment for me.

I cannot explain what compelled me to keep up the struggle, but for eight weeks I was tenacious. I pleaded with teams of doctors from two major Boston hospitals to consider the procedure for me, and while doing so, discovered (as would be the case later on) that the knowledge I had acquired made the doctors more open to carrying on a dialogue with me. I think the doctors were swayed by my determination to have this particular protocol performed and encouraged by all the research that I had done. Most important, I was an appropriate candidate for this surgery. My cancer had not spread to the lymph nodes, or outside the lung area. Finally, my insistence paid off, and the surgery modeling the New York protocol was approved by the hospital medical board.

Then, after all the expended effort and diligent planning, there was a snag. On the evening before the big day, I called my doctor's office to check in one last time on the final coordinated plan. It was the kind of routine call I've always made. Actually, the nurse informed me, the key oncologist was in California at a conference. He wouldn't be back in time to pour the drugs into my lungs. My heart sank. "No need to worry," she said, the surgery would go on. Then she hung up the phone.

Oh no! I thought. I would not consent to the altered plan. The more I thought about it, the more certain I felt. After all that preparation and planning, I wanted it to be right. I called back the doctor's office to postpone the operation.

Fortunately, my oncologist concurred and two weeks later when he returned to Boston, the surgery was performed. I became the first patient to receive this treatment at Brigham and Women's Hospital.

With each step I learned how to trust and listen to my inner voice. "What lies behind us and what lies before us," wrote Oliver Wendell Holmes, "are tiny matters compared to what lies *within* us." Becoming educated and being assertive helped me feel more in control of my destiny and, in turn, allowed the healing process to unfold.

Attitude *matters*. Comparative studies show markedly different outcomes between groups of patients with the same cancer and similar age and socioeconomic backgrounds. Those who stayed strong and positive in the face of their illness, who were actively involved in their treatment, and committed to getting well, had longer survival rates than those who were passive, responded compliantly to what the doctors told them, or never thought to challenge the grim statistics.

In July 1982 the well-known scientist and writer Stephen Jay Gould was diagnosed with *abdominal* mesothelioma and faced a situation much like mine. A computer searched yielded the stomach-punching conclusion that his disease was incurable and that, statistically, he could expect a "median mortality" of only eight months after diagnosis. In other words, he would likely die within eight months.

But Gould's temperament and professional training told him there was another way to interpret the data—that this so called "median" rate also meant that half the people diagnosed with mesothelioma would live *longer*—some, perhaps, much longer. In classic "is the glass half empty or half full" style, Gould read on, looking behind the hard numbers for statistical variation and distribution: what circumstances might allow mesothelioma patients like himself to survive longer, and for how much longer might that be?

What Gould discovered was that he possessed every one of the characteristics the studies indicated should confer a probability of longer life—relative youth, early diagnosis, first-rate treatment, a confident and optimistic attitude. And while Gould's analysis of the statistical literature *promised* nothing, it gave him the precious gifts of hope and time, to think, plan, and fight. About two decades later, Stephen Jay Gould is very much, and gratefully alive.

In their book *Remarkable Recovery*, Caryle Hirshberg and Marc Ian Barasch ask why some people with deadly cancers, and against all odds, get well. They conclude it is because

> These people had the quality of *congruence*. In the midst of crisis they discovered a way to be deeply true to themselves, by manifesting behaviors from the roots of their being. These unlikely survivors had strong connections with others and a few profound nurturing relationships. These factors—a different set for each person—seemed to "jump start" the healing response.

When I went through my cancer experience, I remember the doctor saying to me, "You must have goals. Set goals that are reachable now; set goals that are reachable down the road." Those words stayed with me and made a lasting impression. So throughout my ordeal, I set goals, goals for trips I would take, for projects I wanted to do, for planning dinner parties, for connecting with far away friends, for changing my diet "when" I felt better . . . "as" I became better . . . for when I was "all" better. And he was right. Goals are potent tools that empower and can move our energy to a better place.

"The swords of battle are numerous," Stephen Jay Gould reminds us. Jump start your own healing by looking first to your own truth. Draw on your knowledge, draw on your personal reserves, to find reasons to live and reasons to hope. Becoming personally empowered actually can save your life.

After a while you learn the subtle difference
Between holding a hand
And chaining a soul.
And you learn that love doesn't mean leaning
And company doesn't mean security.
And you begin to learn
That kisses aren't compromises
And presents aren't promises.
And you begin to accept your defeats
With your head up and your eyes ahead
With the grace of a woman or a man
Not the grief of a child.

And you learn to build all your roads on today
Because tomorrow's ground is too uncertain for plans
And futures have a way of falling down in midflight.
After a while you learn that even sunshine burns
if you get too much
So you plant your own garden
And decorate your own soul
Instead of waiting for someone to buy you flowers.
And you learn that you really can endure
That you really are strong.
And you really do have worth.
And you learn. And you learn.
With every failure you learn.

—ANONYMOUS

Statistics are the triumph of the quantitative method,
and the quantitative method is the victory
of sterility and death.
—HILAIRE BELLOC

In the midst of winter, I finally learned that there
was in me an invincible summer.
—ALBERT CAMUS

Like the first star . . . each soul is on fire
With the primordial heat . . . of creation . . .
Intended to illuminate what is unique, mysterious, and
miraculous . . . about life itself.
Intended to bring forth; and bless with breathtaking
brilliance
Each person has the power and grace to change the
world . . .
Each is dancing in a universe of profound possibility.
—SUE MILLER HURST,
FACILITATOR OF THE MIT DIALOGUE PROJECT

8

Meditation

From the moment we awake, our minds create an incessant stream of conscious thoughts, like a running river, sometimes racing, sometimes slowed, but never still. Meditation is a respite, a time for inner quiet. It is the process by which we go about deepening our attention and awareness by clearing the mind.

The act of being in a quieted state while focusing on one's breathing allows time for the mind, body, and soul to establish balance. It returns us to a place of stillness inside ourselves, a place that is peaceful and nonjudgmental. In this safe place we may be at ease, no matter how much stress or trauma surrounds us or what has happened in our emotional and physical lives to transform or upset us.

Learning to access this special place inside each of us is key to finding inner balance. Through the technique of meditation we can locate that quiet place inside which centers us and brings us balance and inner peace. When one is facing a life crisis finding this balance becomes even more crucial. That is because more time is needed for quiet, for reflection, and to get the healing energies within our bodies working well. The more we "do" and "go," the more ruffled our minds are by the winds and storms of daily living, the less our bodies are able to relax and our immune systems to fight.

When I first tried meditation I found it difficult to focus and be still. My mind was riding a raft over white water; I could not find calm or even sit for long. My efforts to meditate frustrated me—and at times I felt as though I was trying to recapture some sixties-like state of rapture as an ailing fortysomething. I felt intimidated by the gurus I tried to emulate, who sat so erect for extended periods of sustained stillness. But I also felt conflicted, for I knew that meditating daily could help me. I had read about its positive benefits, and friends and social workers were encouraging me to try it. I believed that through meditation I would find more mental clarity for making decisions.

So after many weeks of guilt-ridden failure, I decided to compromise. Instead of meditating for twenty minutes as I'd been instructed to do, I tried it for three. Making that choice immediately alleviated the pressure I had felt "to do it right." I began to experiment with the basic methods until I found my own creative way. And soon I found that I began to enjoy it—and slowly to feel that wonderful sense of inner calm I'd hoped for. When I stopped worrying about technique, I stopped feeling frustrated. I simply felt better.

I was reassured later by several enlightened teachers that the meditation process varies for each individual. There is no right way. It can be done for fifty minutes or for fifty seconds. It can be practiced while sitting on the floor crossed-legged or in a chair, while reclining, standing, or walking; to music or in silence, with a timing device or not. And despite its roots in ancient Buddhism, meditation is a practice that need not conflict with any religious beliefs.

I relished this new sense of freedom. Giving myself permission to "do my own thing" allowed me to establish a daily ritual. Meditation books and instructional tapes offer varying but valid instruction. While techniques differ, I found that meditating each day at the same time and when possible in the same location works best for me. I do enjoy meditating to music, and that can range from chamber music and piano compositions by Gershwin. A special favorite of mine consists of soft flute music and is called *Solitude: Rocky Mountain Suite*. Here is what I do:

My Personal Meditation

I sit in a comfortable position with my head and neck erect and my shoulders relaxed. I feel my spine being supported.

I place my hands comfortably in my lap with my palms open. I loosen clothing that is too tight.

I now allow my eyes to close slightly. I begin to focus on each breath. I feel my belly gently expanding with each in-breath and receding with each out-breath. I feel the tension leaving my shoulders, neck, and entire being as it becomes more and more relaxed. Now I focus on my nostrils as the breath passes through them, back and forth.

When thoughts arise, I notice them and let them go. I do not examine them, I simply acknowledge they are there and send them off, a friendly escort to the border of my being. If sensations appear in my body, I notice them and let them go, too. Each time my attention wanders off, as often happens, I bring my attention back to my breath. I feel the breath moving into my body, through my chest, down to my arms, legs, and toes. I notice my feelings, but do not pursue or reject them. I see only what is here in this moment and let myself just be. I work at maintaining my awareness as by breath moves in and out of my body.

When I am ready, I allow my eyes to open gradually and warm myself to the world around. My relaxed state deepens the more often I meditate.

I rise refreshed to greet the day.

The rich sense of well-being meditation gives me is widely supported by clinical research. Over thirty years ago, Dr. Herbert Benson used the phrase "relaxation response" to describe the improved heart and respiratory rates and lowered blood pressure that were attributable to meditation.

More recently, a research study looked at the effect of meditation on a general group of people and found after nine weeks that the actual brain chemistry of the meditators had changed. It was also noted their systems contained more antibodies. Still other studies have suggested that people who meditate heal faster and experience fewer stress-related ailments such as muscle tension and headaches. And meditation has also been shown to alleviate the suffering associated with chronic pain.

Many people ask me about using a mantra such as a word or phrase during the meditation practice. I generally don't, although when I was at my sickest I remember a few sleepless nights, meditating in bed as I sought to quiet myself. Somewhere the words of the AA mantra, "Let go and let God," came into my consciousness. I repeated those words continually into the early hours of the dawn when I tried to focus my mind in meditation during such moments.

Mindfulness

If meditation can be thought of as deliberately emptying the mind to replenish our awareness, mindfulness is its reverse. The Vietnamese monk Thich Nhat Hahn has called mindfulness "the miracle by which we call back in a flash our dispersed mind and restore it to wholeness."

Mindfulness may also be seen as another form of meditation as both are really about taking time to be in the moment. Whenever I stop to pause and reflect and bring my seeking mind to a stop, I conversely revitalize myself. I feel more empowered and in harmony with the world around me and can respond purposefully to each unique moment. When we are more fully awake in our lives, we are in turn closer to our own unique source. This awakened state helps us eliminate stress and strengthen our ability to heal.

Becoming *mindful* can make life simpler. My sunroom looks out on to a saltwater marsh and I relish watching the seasons slowly change. From my window I watch the greenness of the tall blades of grass fade into tones of ocher and tan. I observe the jagged ice formations crusting along the water's edge. I spot an occasional deer leaping through the snow or a stark white swan gracefully floating by. I catch the pond's reflection of the sinking sun as it melts into the graying sky. And I listen to the howling winds rip through my pear trees, making my doors creak. I connect with flowers in my garden, feel the breeze against my face, and always stop to hear the laughter of neighboring children at play.

I am grateful to have a beach house that is in such a beautiful setting. Nature's beauty, however, can be found all around us. When spending weeks in the hospital, I would always find an open courtyard with a bench or a piece of lawn. Just hearing the birds sing and taking in the fresh air were invigorating.

City parks can also offer a place to quiet the mind, sit amid the trees, and smell the earth beneath us. Sometimes I go to a local park with a sandwich and watch life moving around me: the squirrels scampering for pine cones, the breeze blowing the crisp leaves over the pavement, and the cloud formations as they change in the sky. Just walking outdoors or sitting on a front stoop can be all it takes to refresh ourselves.

My favorite mindful practice takes place when I eat lunch out on my deck. First I sit quietly before the food in front of me and take several deep breaths. I become fully conscious of the wondrous gifts surrounding me: the swaying marsh grass, the light reflecting over the saltwater pond, the melodious call of the nesting heron, the baby ducks who come to nibble on the overflow from the bird feeder. As I take my first bite, I begin the process of appreciation. I focus on where the food originated, first from seed to full-grown plant, then getting to market. I offer silent grace.

Next I savor each taste, becoming mindful of the sensations in my mouth. I stop consciously between bites to focus on my breath. I allow myself to become fully immersed in the glory of the fresh ocean air. And as I conclude the meal, I note how revitalized I feel.

During my convalescence, mindfulness taught me a new way of seeing. Applying this practice has opened my consciousness to new gardens within.

Ask! Knock, but don't let anyone sell you
anything . . . for your treasure house is within.
It contains all you will ever need.
—HUI HAI, ZEN MASTER

Mindfulness is about being fully aware in our lives. It is about perceiving the exquisite vividness of each moment. When we feel more alive we gain immediate access to our own inner resources for coping effectively with stress.

—JON KABAT-ZINN,
WHEREVER YOU GO, THERE YOU ARE

In the silence of my meditation, I receive guidance and direction. I am filled with all the power I need to take my next step.

—RUTH FISHEL, *TIME FOR JOY*

Silence was the first prayer I learned to trust.

—PATRICIA HAMPL, *VIRGIN TIME*

9

Visualization

The ability to conjure healthy images in one's mind as a means to stimulate positive physical responses in both our body and emotions is one of the more potent weapons we have in aiding our recovery. Visualization allows us to *reframe* our cancer, to impose a visual framework of our own making on the direction of our healing. When we recruit our imagination to create mental pictures, we are responding proactively to illness by providing a powerful focus around which our emotional, spiritual, and physical energies can rally. Visualization and guided imagery (a related technique) are now widely accepted as effective adjunctive therapies in cancer treatment. I practiced visualization regularly.

The power of imagery in the practice of medicine has a long history going back to the ancient Greeks, thirteenth-century Buddhists, and native cultures around the world. Imagination is more powerful than knowledge, Albert Einstein said. When we work with imagery we are going deep inside ourselves to shape the outcome of our treatment. Just how this physiological process works to mobilize the immune system is unclear, although researchers speculate it proceeds from the understanding that human beings function according to their expectations. Our belief system can have a powerful effect on our health. We expect that summer days will be hot and the sun radiant. So we dress in light clothes and plan a day at the pool. We expect Friday to be followed by Saturday, and our weekend body clocks therefore know to "let down" just as they know to prepare for a more accelerated pace come Monday morning.

When we "visualize" our expectations, we are extending this natural process of programming our body to do what the mind expects of it. Whatever pictorial trigger our mind selects sets up a series of self-regulating inner mechanisms that accept the image as a course of action to be implemented so the desired outcome is obtained.

Dr. Michael Samuels in his book *Healing with the Mind's Eye* was one of the first to recount how a mere thought held in the mind can decrease blood pressure or stimulate the immune system. It is possible, he wrote, to trace a physiological pathway in which this occurs, as visual images create an "excitation of nerve cells which affects the functioning of organs in the body. Although this sounds simple, the process is incredibly complex and has taken years to document." Subsequent studies have reported that patients who used visualization techniques after chemotherapy infusion felt less anxiety, nausea, and depression than control groups who did not. And researchers measuring natural killer cell activity in breast cancer patients over an eighteen-month period found significant effects in improved responsiveness.

I was familiar with the new field of psycho-neuro-immunology and the profound influence the mind/body connection played in overcoming illness. Even during times when I was discouraged, I continually reminded myself that imagery work had value and I must not discount it.

Whenever I could I would begin a brief meditation and take a few deep breaths to relax and focus my concentration. I directed my attention to the part of my body where the cancer was located and envisioned the white fighter cells engulfing the bad cells in my system and destroying them. Then I pictured the cancer leaving my body through natural processes. I imagined my internal organs returning to their natural pink color, healthy again. I repeated this visualization every day. This useful technique became an invaluable lifeline throughout my journey. In time, I expanded upon it and developed my own formal program, which I now share when I present workshops and counsel others. This visualization exercise in its entirety is presented in the next chapter. (See page 63.)

While lying for endless hours in the claustrophobia-inducing tunnels of hospital MRI machines, I made use of a special visualization. I allowed my mind to turn the ear-blasting banging of the machine into the visualized imagery of *hovering angels hammering at my tumor with golden axes*. Chip by chip, piece by piece, I envisioned my tumor decreasing in size.

By doing so I practiced replacing my terror with *potent imagery*. I could feel the exhilaration travel through my bones. Determined to transform my fright, I also wanted to make my time—all of it—count. Sometimes, I envisioned by body enveloped in a white vaporous light. When my mind wandered, I'd bring back the healing light and flash on a joyful memory. I'd hold the memory in my mind's eye like a freeze frame for several moments, so that each cell in my body could absorb the elation I consciously triggered.

Other times I'd redecorate my living room. I'd move the sofa, change the window treatment, reposition the television. Then I might redesign my whole house. I believed that these glistening moments released endorphins into my system, natural fighter chemicals boosting the immune response that would help me get well again. According to the neurobiologist Dr. Candace Pert, the cells in our body respond to our emotional states. When fear arises, our pancreas or liver cells, in fact *all our cells*, pick up on that negative emotion, just as they are nourished by the positive emotions we experience. By using mental imagery to activate joy, I was using my mind and body to help myself heal.

Soon my visualizations became more and more intense and I actually began to feel hopeful. The time passed quickly lying in those massive machines, for I had work to do! I continually used my mind. When the technicians finally rolled me out of that tight steel cave, I had cramped extremities but felt exhilarated.

Accessing our inner resources can maximize our ability to surge forward. Recruit your imaginative power and create your own positive expectations. Make your visualizations vivid, full of detail, and rich with *sensory* images. The stronger and more personally resonant they are, the better the job they do of focusing your energy. Draw on the military imagery of a general leading the charge or on musical images by chasing away your cancer cells with loud cymbals or a *Star Wars* laser. Enlist the animal world by imagining a pride of lions or a swarm of angry bees massed for attack. Think of Roman gladiators or bands of angels—God's "warriors"—all poised to assault and defeat your disease. By using visualization you are calling upon your best defense—your healing power from within.

....

Ultimately, human intentionality is the most powerful evolutionary force on this planet.
—GEORGE LEONARD, *THE LIFE WE ARE GIVEN*,
(WITH MICHAEL MURPHY)

....

10

Creating a
Personal Tape

Preparing for each of my operations (there were two extensive exploratory surgeries prior to my major surgery) and facing the unknown left me feeling tremendous anxiety and fear. Having never experienced major surgery, I was terrified of the postoperative pain. I was frightened about the aggressive chemotherapy that I would undergo, about the months of debilitation I faced, about the grave prognosis that followed me everywhere. I realized I needed to approach the ordeal with a certain inner quiet. I decided to create a relaxation tape *using my own voice*.

There is something about hearing the sound of my own voice that has always resonated to me. I knew that if I could talk to myself I could find calm more easily than I could listening to an instructional meditation tape with somebody else's words. Somebody else was not *me*. As with snowflakes or the boughs of trees, where no two are ever alike, nature produces individuals, and individuality is in our natures.

In creating my tape I chose healing thoughts that inspired me, meditative reflections that would ease and uplift, and guiding words that would steer me through the darkness ahead. The tape included:

- Convincing thoughts repeating that the harsh medical protocol was necessary for my recovery
- Empowering words that emphasized the importance of being relaxed
- Talking to my body to convince it I could tolerate the postsurgical pain and chemotherapy-induced discomfort
- Vocalizing my fears and instructing them to go away
- Affirming words reminding me "I will make it through"
- Asking a higher power for increased strength to cope with what was ahead
- Reinforcing messages that I would do my very best and leave the rest in the hands of the Divine

I took time to gather the positive words that ended up on my tape. I remember the days of sipping tea in my sunroom looking through books of poetry and prayer, some from my bookshelf and some from my own written collection, with my stereo playing everything from Vivaldi to the Boston Pops. These precious moments of peace are warm memories, for the preparation process itself was restorative.

In putting my tape together, I wanted to create an aural collage of written prayers, literary excerpts, musical selections, and motivational sayings that were personally compelling. In looking for just the right words, I tried to be eclectic. I borrowed and bent and sought to keep the tone informal. After several days, when my searching and synthesizing were completed, I began my tape to the accompaniment of Mozart's *Piano Sonata in A Minor* (K.310) and *String Quartet in D Major* (K.575).

The tape I made was a patchwork of meditation, motivation, memory, and message. I spoke of things that stirred me and ignited my spirit—of straw brooms sweeping through my insides pushing away the cancer; of dancing in ballet slippers as a child in our backyard and the freedom and joy I felt; of my intention to be whole and healthy again. These recorded words were the last thing I heard each time I was taken by gurney to the operating room. Once I was out of recovery, I played my tape every day while I was in the hospital and regularly after I returned home.

I found the power of this tape was in hearing my own voice steadying my nerves, driving me on, directing my own body cells toward healing. Not everyone is comfortable hearing her own voice. If that's the case, prepare a script and ask someone close to you to record your tape for you. You may also want to try to include words of love from family and friends. The voice of a friend giving you a forceful, motivational message or a child's voice saying "I love you" can bring you confidence and strength during weak moments.

In recording your tape, plan to devote one side to the visualization processes described in the previous chapter. By opening your tape with a meditation you quiet the body and are prepared to receive the empowering energy of your affirming thoughts. Mental imagery—memories of camping trips, family vacations, holiday dinners, country scenes— will bring back joy and prompt endorphin release. Summoning cancer-fighting imagery like laser beams and hot liquid gold can zap and rid the body of malignant tissue. The imagery of rejuvenation and health will bring you the reality.

I discovered there is something truly magical about listening to the repetitive sound of one's own voice. Many long months later, just after my final chemo, with radiation still in store, I attended an outdoor concert with my family. I was so moved by what happened that evening I was compelled to describe it on my tape. I spoke of how the *1812 Overture* played during a Fourth of July fireworks display brought an enormous rush of gratitude. I could actually feel the final purging of cancer cells from my body. I knew my body cells were truly responding to the potent words I played daily and absorbing their message. As the audience cheered the soaring flashes of light, I imagined they were cheering for me, for my freedom from this disease.

After a full year of listening to my cancer tape I decided to take a break. I put a colorful label on it with a drawing of a smiling dinosaur and put the cassette into an old shoe box under my bed. Not wanting to write the actual word, I wrote "Canser Tape" on the label. Later on, I made a new tape with a fresh set of affirmations and used more upbeat music. This time, I included the Gloria Gaynor anthem "I Will Survive," along with some Judy Collins folk songs. I spent time allowing myself to feel gratitude for having come through the year's ordeal and continually envisioned my body "whole, healthy, and perfect." Those words became my postsurgical mantra. And I added a few goals I wanted to achieve, such as spending time designing new greeting cards, working on a book of personal memories, and planning a mini-getaway with my husband to a special inn in the Berkshire Mountains. The next year, I made another tape.

Each of my tapes were inspiring and played a strong role in my continued recovery. But of all the tapes I made, none was more powerful than the original "Canser Tape." My words were stronger, my determination unbeatable. That tape traveled with me everywhere through my journey. It was the map that guided me home.

Creating a Visualization Tape

As my recovery progressed, I drew on diverse sources to build upon the visualization techniques that had already taken me so far. With practice I found that meditation came easier and my imaging grew stronger. I became more focused in my daily living and more confident about dealing with the unknowns of my disease. I knew that my visualization work was profoundly affecting my physical, emotional, and spiritual health. Then I began to incorporate my new findings and collected insights into a more structured program that I practiced every day. I blended it with a special meditation session, added three deliberately chosen visualization scenarios, and concluded it with a series of carefully selected prayers and affirmations. I then spoke into a pocket recorder and made an empowering tape. Again, hearing my own voice and directing my body cells became an extraordinary tool in my healing.

Here is a description of the steps in making your own visualization tape.

Step One: Meditation. Access your healing system by beginning to focus intently on your breathing. Relax your shoulders; place your hands comfortably in your lap with your palms open to allow universal energy to come through. Notice how your belly expands on each in-breath and gently recedes on each out-breath. Try to fully experience each breath as it enters in and out of your nostrils. As your mind wanders acknowledge any scattered thoughts and let them go. Always bring your attention back to your breath.

By breathing deeply, you are allowing more oxygen to travel through your system. The oxygen we take in enlarges the passages into our brain, and increases the circulatory pathways that will carry your visualized expectations from your mind to each organ in your body.

As you feel the tension leaving, go to that special place inside where there is full calm, that inner place where you can always just go to "be." Enter this sacred place acknowledging that you have the power within you to boost your immune system. Stay in this focused meditation for several minutes on your tape. Always leave pauses, speaking no words, for a deeper relaxation.

Step Two: Reflection. Look back on your life as if you were watching a rolling movie reel. Try to remember a time, a place, a special moment where you felt totally joyful, fully embraced with love and connection to others, perhaps your daughter's wedding.

Recall that experience and enrich it with sensory detail relating to sound, touch, taste, sight, and smell. Remember the beautiful dress your daughter wore and the expression on her face as she made her vows. Notice the warm glow of candlelight as you sat amid the colorful table settings and the fragrance in the air from the flower bouquets. Hear the chiming champagne glasses touching as the wedding toast is given. (If you have trouble resurrecting this image, avoid frustration and "sneak up" on it slowly. Let your mind return to the early preparations of getting ready for the day, from rising that morning through the many steps you took to get to the ceremony. When you are ready, gently step inside the scene.)

Feel the heightened energy run through you as you envision yourself in this glorious place. Feel the love surrounding you from family and friends. Stay in that moment and hold the magic, again for several minutes. The joyous emotions you are experiencing now are releasing endorphins from your brain, a morphine-like substance that enables your body to boost your immune system and fight harder. Imagine you are holding a camera. Snap a photo of this moment in your mind. See it and let it go.

Relax your body and bring your attention back to your breath to restore balance again. Know that you are still in a peaceful but powerful place inside yourself, a place where you have just strengthened your ability to help yourself and enhance your immune system.

Step Three: The Cancer Scene. Imagine now with all your power that you have the ability to go inside your body with your mind. Go boldly up to that area where you see the cancer cells. Describe to yourself what they look like, their shape, color, texture, and size. Are they tiny dark spots? Jelly bean– or amoeba-shaped? Marble-size globules or microscopic dots? Be creative.

Imagine that you have the full power to eradicate these cells, one by one. Envision the instrument that you are going to take inside your body to do this. Some people will suction out their unwanted cells with a micro-vacuum cleaner; some envision using a laser beam or a wand with golden fire. Some use a mini-shovel. Be aggressive and make your choice something that feels right for you.

Step Four: Elimination. As you begin the process of removing these cells, one by one, see each individual cell being destroyed. Be meticulous, be thorough. Take all the time you need to get the job done. When all the cells have been eradicated, it is very important to expel them from your body. Imagine being in the shower washing the cells off. Think about brushing your teeth each morning and spitting out the cells with toothpaste and saliva. See them leaving your body through your pores or in a liquid stream from your own natural urination process. Choose one that works for you. Envisioning a natural bodily process of elimination triggers the daily reinforcement of your behavior and strengthens your visualization. Watch the cells leave your body. They are gone with the flush of a toilet. They are no longer inside you.

Step Five: Rejuvenation. Return to your deep and focused breathing. See your body tissues whole, healthy, pink, and clean. Hold this image of your internal health for several minutes. As you take a moment to center yourself, know that you have used your body's innate healing ability to help guide you back to health.

With your cancer scene completed and inner health and harmony restored, you may want to add another joyful reflection to your tape, as in Step Two—graduation day, a fishing trip, a hike in the mountains, lying on a beach, or anything that strikes a chord. Always end the scene by reaffirming that you have the power to help your immune system.

Conclude your visualization tape by now adding meaningful affirmations. Select thoughts that move you and open your heart. Affirm the power within by using motivating words and prayer that resonate with your own being. (Note: Adding music in the background is a personal choice. I find it enhances the program.)

The initial mystery that attends any journey is:
how did the traveler reach his starting point
in the first place?

—LOUISE BOGAN,
JOURNEY AROUND MY ROOM

11

Book of

Affirmations

I purchased a colorful cloth book with blank pages and began to fill it with quotations, poetry, and inspirational thoughts I came across. Reading a line after my morning meditation gave me an emotional lift. I added to the book whenever I found something meaningful. My book became a patchwork, drawing together varied and multitudinous voices in the cause of my own healing. When I began composing affirmations of my own, my book became even more of a powerful tool for healing.

Affirmations are clear, straightforward statements of positive expectation. They are most helpful when written in the present tense and are highly effective in creating a *concentrated intentionality* to change our functioning in a beneficial way. They build confidence. Unlike journal writing, which expansively examines one's own thoughts, emotions, and reflections, affirmations are short and directed. One is generally descriptive; the other prescriptive. Both are transformative.

Even on the days I felt depleted I forced myself to read a few lines of motivational thoughts. It has been shown that positive stimuli can induce the brain to produce its own immune-enhancing endorphins. Words carry power; and by reading upbeat and motivating messages, I was enabling my body to release these natural chemicals.

Words—all words—have the ability to change our thought patterns and can open new pathways toward healing. It doesn't matter whether they are written by you or someone else. I gathered many affirmations from my reading. Accumulating them gave me a feeling of security, as though if I gathered enough of them I would cross over some magical line and arrive on the safe side. Whenever I would dip in and out of my collection I always felt as though I were drinking from the strong waters of health.

I put some of my favorite affirmations onto my personal tape. I also used four-x-six-inch index cards as flash cards. I carried these in a packet in my purse or jacket everywhere I went so I could read them when I had a few moments, in the physician's office while waiting to be seen or while standing in line at the pharmacy. Even the briefest reinforcement works, helping to program the brain to think differently.

Here is an actual page taken from my affirmation book:

I am whole, healthy, and healed.

I embrace the mystery of each new dawn.

No unwanted cells will ever grow in me again.
My immune system is powerful and can fight off
diseases. I love my immune system!

Straw brooms are sweeping through my insides
pushing out the cancer cells and fearful thoughts.
I see my organs turning pink and clean.

I am still awed by a single line I wrote and double-underlined in hot pink marker. It reads:

I WILL LIVE A LONG LIFE . . . I WILL BEAT ALL
ODDS!

With every year of health, my collection of affirmations continues to build. After my book was filled with words, I began another. My home is where my books of affirmation are.

All is well and all is well and all
manner of things are well.
—JULIAN OF NORWICH

My barn having burnt down,
I can see the moon.
—ANONYMOUS

You gain strength, courage and confidence
by every experience in which you really stop
to look fear in the face . . . You must do the
things you think you cannot do.
—ELEANOR ROOSEVELT

12

Reaching Out

When one is caught in the midst of an intense battle for one's life, the mundane details of everyday living can feel overwhelming. Yet errands must be run, meals prepared, laundry done, bills paid. You are in no shape to do it by yourself. Learning to reach out to others allowed me to luxuriate in the process of being "supported" while my body took time to heal.

After hearing my grave diagnosis, my loved ones called continually. Some froze, tongue-tied and frightened, unable to find the sustaining words they wanted to convey.

But action is another expression of caring. "I wish there was something I could do." many said almost reflexively. There was. As I came to accept their offers of help, these friends became a lifeline, each generous act a link in a process that got me through my ordeal.

I found that people appreciate direction regarding how they can best serve. My guidance made them feel comfortable and needed. I learned to be specific about my needs. Friends shopped for groceries, went to the drugstore, drove me to the hospital and to doctor visits, picked up books and tapes from the library, dropped off clothes at the cleaner. After chemo, my husband asked a friend to roast a turkey: it was in the oven when we came home.

We created a shift arrangement with neighbors and friends to stay with me so Ralph could go to work. Neighbors had keys to the house and sometimes we would come home from a medical appointment to find homemade brownies or a warm meal waiting. Later, members of my women's group and book club circulated a sign-up sheet for volunteers to take me back and forth from radiation.

The outpouring of support inspired me and speeded my recovery. The hardest part was, after the initial flurry of concerned phone calls dropped off, learning to ask. That I was able to muster the necessary dignity and grace to do so never made it easier. Every time I reached out to ask for help, a piece of me crumbled inside. Still, I learned to be skilled at it, and the ready generosity of the circle of friends and family who assisted me is something I'll never forget.

If asking is difficult for you, or if the network of helpers available to you is limited, check to see what resources and services exist where you live. Many communities have programs where volunteers provide meals and perform errands for families in crisis. Their efforts are confidential. Your place of worship will very likely have something comparable, too.

In addition to riding with friends to morning radiation appointments each day, I discovered that many localities provide free rides to hospitals from a staff of generous volunteers. In my case the volunteer driver service offered by the local branch of the American Cancer Society was a tremendous help. I was given the names of drivers in my area who donated their time to transport cancer patients to medical appointments.

I was deeply touched by these extraordinary people who gave their time to deliver me safely to each appointment. I remember how comforting it was to chat with these drivers about mundane things during the ride. Very often, they would share with me their personal stories, and this always had a calming effect on me. Most of them had family members who had had cancer and understood the anxiety and stress I was feeling when I made my way to even the most routine of visits.

Cancer is a prolonged fight, and so if you have children at home, you will need to reach out for help with the normal routines of child care, homework, meal preparation, and carpooling. One woman battling breast cancer while raising three small children called upon "her angels"— three close women friends—and asked each to "buddy up" with one of her children as a surrogate and "special friend"; a cheerleader and confidant available for that one child during the time when Mom was too sick and didn't have the energy to attend school plays, soccer games, or even cuddle up for a heart-to-heart.

I continually searched for ways to show my appreciation and to give back even when I wasn't feeling well and there was little I could do. When I could, I would spend afternoons in bed painting flower motifs or cutting up stacks of recycled birthday cards. I would take sections of the card designs and cut them into rectangular shapes. Then after putting a hole punch in the corner, I would insert fanciful ribbons which I would tie or curl. On the reverse side of the homemade card I would write a message of appreciation or gratitude to the person who had come by or had done something to help us. When I felt better, I would pick a flower from my garden and tie one of my little notes around it and give it to the friend who was dropping off groceries or driving me that day. Shortly after my treatment ended, my husband and I invited each of my volunteer drivers to a restaurant of their choice for an appreciation dinner. It felt good to say thanks!

We are each of us angels with only one wing.
We can fly only by embracing each other.
—LUCIANO DE CRESCENZO

The spirit will emerge through the lives of ordinary people who will hear a call and answer in extraordinary ways.

—MOTHER TERESA

Fragrance always stays in the hand that gives the rose.

—ANONYMOUS

13

Dealing with Well-Wishers

I was buoyed by the outpouring of concern from my circle of friends and family. Never had friends seemed more important. "My friends are my estate," as Emily Dickinson wrote. Yet when dealing with the overwhelming number of well-wishers, I consciously worked at not dwelling on myself. I found the continual retelling of my story to be enormously draining, even as I understood my visitors' questions and expressions of interest reflected genuine concern. Finally, I decided to be candid and explain to people that "I couldn't talk about it much."

Well-meaning friends and family are not always aware of the emotional exhaustion caused by repeating a scenario again and again. Discussing the details forced me to mentally relive the frightening drama at a time when my emotions and energy were raw and compromised. During convalescence you need to go ahead and not back, to cleanse yourself of the memory of your illness, just as your body is now cleansed. When asked to tell my story, I learned to be informative but brief.

During my weakest times, I graciously accepted friends' offers to return the many phone calls that kept coming in. Concerned supporters wanted to keep up with my progress. By assigning a friend the task of telephone duty to relay a quick report on how I was doing, my family and I were able to conserve time and energy. Today I would have used my e-mail "buddy list" to post such health updates. It is an efficient, user-friendly way to keep your circle close. Above all, I wanted to allow my friends and family to participate in my healing, and understood their need to feel a part of what was happening.

I have always had a strong interest in other people. I made a concerted effort to hear about my visitors' lives and interests. Dwelling on one's pain for an extended length of time can stifle the natural flow of healing. I knew it was important to honor the recovery process and to use the tools that can help our bodies heal. Getting out of myself became important. To do this I concentrated intently on their stories and practiced what is known as active listening, a form of focused listening that I used to divert me from my own suffering.

Active listening also became a way of engaging my callers and helping them enjoy our time together. I often found visitors terribly self-conscious with me. On the one hand, they didn't want to make me feel bad by asking about my situation; nor did they want to make me feel left out by talking too enthusiastically about their travels and triumphs. It wasn't unusual for some of them to respond to that most innocuous of social niceties, "How are you?" with an apology.

I like "active" listening because it signals an openness to another's message. So when my friends shared their experiences, by the expression on my face or by nodding my head or by restating the feelings I was hearing from them in my own words, I could keep the conversation going. Active listening not only put my visitors at ease—easing the sometimes subtle discomfort between us—but also allowed me to feel part of them for a while at a critical time when I was so overwhelmed with fear and pain. The feeling of connection, of participation in life's vivid flow, was profound.

During this time I continued my ritual of making special homemade cards for each friend's birthday. I remember the extreme exhaustion I felt whenever the calendar reminded me another occasion was approaching. Still I managed to complete each project with enough time so it would arrive by the right date. I am not sure why I pushed myself to continue this practice, but in reflection it seems it was an instinctual method that again helped me *get out of myself*. In the process I discovered that *my giving gave healing back*. Giving pleasure brings joy and in turn can enhance your immune system.

How to Use Active Listening

Active listening is a simple but powerful communication tool where the receiver learns to communicate an attitude of empathetic understanding to the person he is engaged in conversation with. It involves suspending one's own thoughts in order to respond to the sender's message. While not difficult to learn, good active listening requires practice. The receiver only needs to restate, in his own language, his impression of the sender's words. Active listening does not attempt to disguise feelings. It is, instead, a vehicle for encouraging the open expression of feelings. This technique can bring people closer and let the speaking person feel he is being really heard. Example:

> DONNA: I am afraid to go to the doctor this morning for those tests.
> DAVE: You are feeling fearful today.
> DONNA: Yes, I have knots in my stomach.

DAVE: You are feeling tense and are hesitant about going.

DONNA: Yes, I am. I know I have to go. Let's get in the car.

DAVE: You have decided to have the tests.

DONNA: I have. Thanks, Dave. It's so hard for me. I really appreciate your just listening.

14

Medication

Drugs that help with pain management following surgery and the nausea that often accompanies chemotherapy are important pieces of the recovery process.

In the hospital following both my major surgeries, I was given the use of a morphine pump, which allowed me to take charge of administering my own pain medication. The pump is computer-programmed with a dosage determined by the type of surgery and the degree of pain anticipated to result. It has specific parameters and an automatic shutoff that is tightly controlled after the designated amount is allotted.

Intravenous lines connected to my veins were hooked up to the pump, a rolling machine on a pole that stood next to my bedside. When the pain became unbearable I pushed a button that immediately released the narcotic into my bloodstream. The use of this device gave me a sense of independence, allowing me to feel in command of my body, rather than a nurse or doctor, during my postsurgical convalescence. Studies show that this method of pain control is most effective.

It is important to be aware of the types of medications and techniques a hospital offers to make a patient more comfortable. I was fortunate to be in a hospital that made the morphine pump available. Do check ahead to see what accommodations your hospital provides.

After leaving the hospital, I experienced periods of arduous pain as my body continued to mend from the surgery. Even the anesthesia lingered in my system, an aftereffect causing me extreme continuous nausea for six to eight weeks. I discovered there is a wide choice of natural or synthetic medications available to control pain and to help reduce nausea, but they can induce side effects such as stomach upset and lethargy. I have always been drug sensitive and found that sometimes my reactions to the medications I was given upon discharge were worse than the original discomfort. One medication actually exacerbated the nausea. After a few days, I decided I wanted to cleanse my system of the drugs I had been given. Other than Ativan, an anti-anxiety medication that I took to help me relax before sleep, I chose to endure the pain and abstain from any medications for the remaining months of my recovery.

I can remember sitting on the edge of my bed, rocking my upper torso while simultaneously rubbing both knees with my palms. The steady motion diverted my focus and eased the postsurgical pain. I also used visualization techniques and listened to soothing music to find relief. When I had more energy, walking outdoors was helpful.

Several months into my recovery, I felt stronger and decided to wean myself from the small dose of Ativan I was taking. I began by cutting one pill in half and taking it every *other* night. Each week I gradually cut back until none were left in the bottle. Although I experienced no adverse side affects, I found it difficult. Soon I began to notice the stress dissipating and I was able to fall asleep without the medication.

With chemotherapy, my nausea returned with a vengeance. Chemotherapy attacks cancer cells as they take in nourishment or when they divide to make new cells. As they do their work, chemotherapy medications do not differentiate between diseased and healthy tissue, which is what produces the much-feared side effects of hair loss (as chemotherapy attacks healthy cells in hair follicles), nausea (healthy cells in the gastrointestinal tract), and extreme fatigue (anemia caused by destroying the red blood cells that give us energy).

Depending on the course of treatment, chemotherapy may be taken in capsule form or through intravenous infusion, performed under in- or outpatient conditions. It may be administered to shrink tumors prior to surgery or radiation or after the tumor has been removed to discourage the growth of new or any remaining cancerous tissue. Treatments are usually given in cycles over a period of months to attack cancer cells at their different life cycle points, which is why the discomfort often associated with this course of treatment may be of long duration.

Each time I had chemotherapy, I stayed in the hospital for three days. The staff offered me medication and suppositories to counteract some of the adverse effects and nausea. Again, not tolerating drugs well, I opted to fight the side effects mostly on my own. I looked to natural herbal therapies like DGL (deglycrhizinated licorice) to strengthen the mucus lining of my stomach and ease upset, as well as green tea, cinnamon tea, and crystallized ginger to fight nausea. (There is also a cinnamon-flavored drink made from slippery elm that eases chemotherapy-related esophageal inflammation.) I did go home with a prescription bottle of yellow marijuana pills thinking that this was pretty cool! After swallowing the first one and experiencing a hallucinogenic out-of-body experience, I realized my drug sensitivity was more pervasive than I had thought, and this "therapy" was not for me either. Feeling out of control was more discomforting to me than the acute nausea.

It is important to recognize that each person has an individual response to chemotherapy and that some patients do amazingly well with it. A new class of antiemetic drugs, known by their brand names Kytril, Zofran, and Anzemet, are also proving effective antinausea therapies. Cancer researchers are working on new chemotherapies that would target only diseased cells. By bypassing healthy cells, chemotherapy patients would experience fewer side effects.

Consult with a hospital nutritionist before and after chemotherapy so you know what kinds of foods you are best likely to tolerate. I was told to eat soft foods and a lot of banana milkshakes. I was reminded to be conscious of vitamin B and to eat red meat at least twice a week to replenish my iron supply. The nutritionist told me to be sure to scrub the skins of fruits and vegetables, as raw, uncooked vegetables can carry bacteria. Because I became temporarily neutropenic (my white blood count was very low from the chemo) I was told not to use a paring knife because even a small cut could cause a severe infection. While I was in chemotherapy and my immune system was still quite compromised, I also was very conscious of staying away from crowds or anyone with colds or infections.

Always check with your doctor regarding dietary restrictions and vitamin use while you are under treatment. Many physicians tell their patients to discontinue the use of antioxidant and vitamin supplements, which may reduce the effectiveness of certain medications they take.

It is important to honor the powerful role drugs play in our convalescence. Each individual's chemistry is unique and each person responds in a different way. Medicines are there to help us and when used properly for the purpose of warding off nausea and pain, the results can be very positive. Discuss with your medical team what options are available to you to ease the transition from surgery to wellness. Using medication appropriately can offer needed comfort and facilitate your healing.

When discussing with your physician the medications you will be taking for pain control, for chemotherapy, and to manage chemotherapy-induced nausea, prepare a list of questions first. You may wish to ask:

- What postoperative drugs will I be given? Will I be permitted to administer this medication directly?
- How long will I be on pain medication?
- What combination of chemotherapy medications will I be taking?
- What are the potential risks associated with this course of treatment?
- How will the drugs be administered (capsule or intravenously)?
- Where will my treatments take place? How long will each last?
- What are the anticipated side effects and for how long will they persist?
- Are there any side effects I should report immediately?
- How will the effectiveness of my chemotherapy be evaluated?
- If tests conclude this protocol is not working for me, what are my options?
- While I am receiving chemotherapy, what can I do to maximize its benefits?

15

Stress Deflection

Trying to sustain an inner calm while in a healing state can be a challenge. You are still emotionally fragile; you have been through so much. You want to maintain the progress you are making in your return to health, yet the normal stresses of daily life go on. There is the stress of feeling more dependent, having to help an aging parent, trying to manage your home or office, keeping finances in order, caring for your children, and maintaining your friendships. And on top of it all, you are dealing with blood counts, radiation, doctor visits, and mortality.

After my surgery, my world continued to implode in ways small and large. Just as my widowed mother was mending from kidney surgery, we learned she had advanced colon cancer. This news, on top of my own critical situation, was devastating. Knowing my mother and I had limited time together, I was determined to move her from her home in upstate New York to Boston so we could spend her last months together. Attempting initially to shield her from our grim diagnoses, and knowing I was in no position to care for her at my house, I secretly searched the Sunday classifieds for a live-in situation and traveled from town to town visiting elder care facilities, at a point when I was thoroughly worn out by the treatments I had just started. In the midst of the hunt, I worried if she would even agree to my plan once the arrangements were made. That my husband and I were going to have to sit her down and eventually tell her the medical facts, mine and hers, weighed heavily on my heart. To this day I thank God she was able to see me, her only child, recovering and doing well when she died.

In addition to this, we were in the process of winterizing our vacation home on Cape Cod so I would be able to go there to relax during my healing. One day I received a panic call from the contractor saying the injection process being used to insulate hadn't worked. The walls in all three bedrooms had cracked. Some had crumbled, leaving bare wood and large holes to the outside. The furniture was full of dust and soot. The contractor claimed the house wasn't properly constructed; we argued back he hadn't been competent. Finally we had to call in another company to repair the job.

Still more months into my recovery, we were faced with an unexpected financial crisis. Suddenly decisions had to be made, legal papers prepared and signed, and we were left in a state of flux. The drama forced us to sell our house and move to the small condo we still owned thirty miles away. Packing boxes, selling furniture, and organizing belongings when I was trying to regain strength felt overwhelming. The chaos never seemed to end.

But I also knew that somehow *my health had to take precedence*. Intuitively I understood what we know is medically true—that stress and negativity are counterproductive to the healing process. In fact, research shows that the body releases cortisol, a natural negative chemical, during periods of stress, and that in abundance this may cause the immune system to break down and physical problems to begin. I knew that if I could not control the stress that is an unavoidable part of living, at least I had the power to regulate the way my body *experienced* it. My life depended on it.

So I learned to deflect stress rather than absorb it. Just as students are taught in medical school to listen but not get too close, stress deflection was my way of keeping my distance from the pain and the negative emotions flying around me from people and situations in my life. It is amazing during crisis how priorities become very clear.

The technique I used centered on the image of a glass prism which I envisioned protectively around me. This glass prism insulated me from the negative emotional content of whatever life was throwing at me. This way I could listen to my husband when he came home each night and shared his challenges of the day; I could listen to my girl-friend talk about a failed romance or a neighbor update me about a troubling political issue in our town. The glass prism prevented me from taking on their stress, yet still allowed me to participate in the world beyond my disease.

This is what I did:

1. As I sat in conversation with someone, taking in information that might be stressful, I would take a deep, cleansing breath. I would envision the glass prism form protectively around me. I saw its walls, I saw it encompassing my body. I saw myself in its center. I saw the glass prism as a layer of safety. I held on to this image.

2. At the same time I maintained my level of alert-ness. I heard what was being said to me, but I pictured the words coming and going, as I watched the pain and upset bounce off the glass walls like bullets, hearing but not letting them penetrate. I would offer my companion very limited responses as I tried not to engage in too much conversation. I would nod my head, raise my eyebrows, and use body language to let him or her know I was listening, but my focus was to protect myself first.

3. And while I listened I silently told myself, over and over, like a mantra, *pull back, pull back,*

Margie; you can only handle your healing at this time. The focus has to be on you now. You must keep yourself together and remain strong. I would say these words over and over in my head. Again and again and again.

4. As I recited this mantra, I continued to focus on my breath, knowing that deep breathing actually moves the oxygen through the body faster, helping me let go of tension and restore balance.

This mindful practice takes discipline and focus yet allows us to remain involved in personal relationships during trying moments or difficult times. It gives us a place of safety when we feel overwhelmed by whatever stress people are bringing to us. And it allows us to respond from a rational place inside rather than coming from a place of upset and agitation. We must remember we have limited capacity when we are ill for taking in unnecessary emotional discomfort. There will be other times in our lives to fully be there for loved ones. But not now. This is a period of *forgivable selfishness*, a time that *will* pass as health improves.

The glass prism technique I used can be adapted to fit your own imagery. You can think of yourself wrapped in your favorite blanket, hidden behind a shield, a bulletproof vest, or something else that will repel flak. You might even imagine yourself climbing into the pilot's seat of a small plane and taking off, flying high above the stress, leaving it behind. Draw on your own imagery, then create a mantra of your own ("I am impenetrable, nothing will harm me").

Wrapping yourself in visualized protection will help you deal with unwelcome intrusions.

······

"The bow always strung . . . will not do."
—GEORGE ELIOT,
MIDDLEMARCH

······

16

Unconditional Love

Aside from dealing with the caustic side effects of chemotherapy, I also had the sudden loss of all my hair, eyelashes, and eyebrows. I struggled with the reactive depression that comes from experiencing this form of trauma. On some days I felt encouraged and on other days quite low. Keeping my spirits up became a major focus of my energies.

During treatment, I received a constant stream of love from friends and family. My husband became accepting of whatever I said or did. He was more patient and helpful than ever before. If I became agitated, he would sit quietly and hold my hand rather than walk out of the room. If I was cold, he would find an extra blanket. Before he left for work he would make sure I had plenty of juices, fruit, and water by my bedside. He would buy me flowers. Friends dropped meals on my doorstep, brought little gifts—poetry books and watercolor art markers—to cheer me, and made themselves available to meet a multitude of my needs each week.

Taking in the abundance of unconditional love made me feel enormously supported and cared for. My husband planned a special surprise for my forty-fourth birthday—a party that caught me completely unaware. He took me out for a sandwich and when we returned home and turned on the lights, fifty friends crouching beside the living room furniture greeted me in song. It was an evening of genuine celebration, as I had just finished my last round of chemotherapy. My body still weakened from the treatment, I fought off the exhaustion as I opened the gifts. I even forgot I hadn't wanted anyone to see me with my stringy wig. The feeling of that transcendent night, and the outpouring of love and generosity that carried me through the many long months and expedited my recovery, is with me still.

The empowerment that comes from receiving love with no boundaries is immeasurable. Asking for unconditional love during your convalescence means being candid and telling loved ones you need them to be more patient, more understanding, more accepting—of your mood swings, your need for quiet in the house, and your need for physical help. Although asking for unconditional love does not always guarantee you'll receive it, it can raise the consciousness of those around you, foster change, and have a dynamic effect on your healing experience. As Karl Menninger once said, "Love cures people, both the ones who give it and the ones who receive it."

The essence of our being is love. Love cannot be hindered by what is merely physical. Therefore, we believe the mind has no limits; nothing is impossible; and all disease is potentially reversible.
—GERALD JAMPOLSKY, M.D.

17

Support Groups

We all tend to feel alone in our suffering. I felt a need to share my feelings with those going through a similar experience and to hear theirs. The social worker from the cancer center where I was being treated gave me information about cancer support groups in my area.

Being a participant in a local support group provided a safe place to really "say it like it is." An immediate kinship developed among our members, a special comfort we could offer each other unlike anyone else. It felt right to be in a place where I would express my deepest concerns. Our meeting became the highlight of my week.

There is a shared understanding in a support group of what it is really like, day to day, to experience the physical and emotional consequences of disease. We would discuss things we didn't or couldn't talk about in social gatherings, or even with our closest friends. Illness is deeply personal territory, and no matter how intimate you are with someone, if that person is healthy, he or she is an outsider. Where else could "How did you lose your last bunch of hair?" spark a vibrant conversation? Where else could you find support and still laugh over the whole horrible experience of becoming bald?

Our group spoke about pain and exchanged valuable information about medications we had found to minimize the discomfort associated with chemotherapy. We talked about the doctors we had seen and who had been kind and gentle and who had been less sensitive and we learned about which hospitals delivered the best services. When we talked about our families we discussed our concerns about not wanting to burden them, our feelings of dependency, our dreams of resuming normal lives. We spoke of the guilt we felt for inconveniencing those we loved and for having their schedules pitch and roll according to the new demands and responsibilities our illness had inflicted on them.

We shared how strange it felt to have our bodies rearranged, reshaped, and raked with scars. We talked about sexual relations, or rather their absence: not only about how asexual we felt, and how our sex drives had gotten lost somewhere between our fear and exhaustion, and perhaps the drying effect chemotherapy has on the skin and mucus membranes, but also the difficulty we had explaining ourselves to our partners. It helped to talk among ourselves about how we had forgotten how to feel feminine and how simply putting on lipstick and a new outfit or going out for a fancy dinner just didn't work. The men discussed how physical weakness made them feel less manly, how something essential felt lost because they could no longer carry a bag of groceries or mow the lawn. Discovering from each other that cancer palpably and inevitably alters relationships not just with spouses or partners but shakes relationships within the entire family helped, too. We told stories of our teenagers who were hesitant to bring their friends home and of younger children who seemed weighed down by the multiple responsibilities—and anxieties—illness thrusts upon them. Our shared stories and experiences allowed us to go beyond our own situations, to see we were not alone, lightening the sense of isolation each of us felt.

The sharing we experienced as a group together made a difference in our emotional outlook. There is nothing as profound as the connection that takes place when like-minded people share the deepest parts of themselves. The benefits are not only emotional, but have physiological implications as well.

A landmark 1989 study by Stanford University psychologist Dr. David Spiegal found that women with advanced breast cancer who attended weekly support groups lived an average of eighteen months longer than those who did not participate in such groups.

Aside from the local support group I joined, I was fortunate to have also enrolled in a six-week program for cancer patients, sponsored by the Deaconess Hospital in Boston, called "The Mind-Body Connection." The program offered a combination of personal sharing and informative lectures from oncologists, nurses, radiation technicians, and social workers. I found both experiences invaluable.

When both groups terminated I helped a friend start a cancer support group on Cape Cod, where I spend half my time each year. That warm crew continues to welcome new members. It is an inspiring group of caring souls who reach out to the community with open hearts. Whenever I can attend I always come away with a renewed sense of what real *giving* is all about.

I encourage you to begin your own group if none exists where you live. Placing a notice on a hospital bulletin board is an effective way to attract members. Speak to a hospital social worker about assisting you in setting up the group; inquire as to whether there is a small meeting room available. Contacting local physicians and mental health professionals to help get out the word may even inspire them to participate in a meeting.

There are many ways to structure a group, but my experience was best when a group of ten to twelve met weekly. We would start by going around the room with each of us sharing something about what had gone on during the week and expressing whatever feelings or fears we had experienced. As we each did our check-in, the members of the group would listen, ask questions, and acknowledge our reactions. By hearing each other's stories and affirming our similar feelings, we built a stronger connection and felt better about ourselves. At the end of the sharing we would introduce a group topic. These might include how we dealt with emotional stress this week; how to bring more joy into our lives; how to deal with our fear; how to get the doctor to call us back; how to learn to ask the right questions. We even discussed the positive effects on our lives that coping with this experience had brought us.

Discussion groups are often more effective if someone is willing to be a facilitator for the group. If no one volunteers, a rotating facilitator may be appointed, so that each week one member takes the role of choosing a topic, overseeing the meeting, and making sure individuals feel included and that each person who wants to speak gets a turn. A designated coleader can be responsible for making phone calls to arrange rides and refreshments.

From time to time, inviting a speaker to join you can be helpful. You can ask someone from your medical team, the hospital staff (such as the patient advocate), or a cancer patient you know who is now doing very well. You can also invite someone from the community who can offer information on nutrition and health, purchasing wigs, or using makeup to give color to your cheeks and to enhance your eyebrows. It is important to strive for a balance of learning and sharing and try to keep the tone as upbeat and positive as possible.

Support for Your Partner

My husband was a vital source of caring, understanding, and support during my recovery. However, the overwhelming load that spouses or partners carry is sometimes taken for granted. The strain on them at this time is enormous. We tend to forget that they are feeling afraid, too. As the author and cancer survivor Betty Rollin has observed, "Disease may score a direct hit on only one member of a family, but shrapnel tears the flesh of the others."

During illness, spouses take on the burden of the caretaker role. Often, there is a reversal of roles. Suddenly a man may be asked to run a household and perform nursing duties, tasks he may never have performed before. For the first time, a woman may have to take over the family finances, replace storm windows, and clean gutters. While all the sympathy and attention seem to be focused on the ill spouse, the caretaker's needs are often overlooked. In a distraught state themselves, they are expected to play a heroic role. Not surprisingly, moodiness, anger, and irritability may set in.

I vividly remember the night two days before my surgery. We had invited close friends in for a small dinner party. My husband, overwhelmed by what was ahead and stressed to the breaking point, decided he did not want to stay. Just before our company was due, he left the house and drove to our home on Cape Cod for a respite. It was difficult for me to be left alone to entertain our good friends, but I knew that what was happening to me was really happening to us. My ordeal was his ordeal, and this was his way of coping: his survival instinct told him at that moment to get out of the path of an avalanche.

We need to realize that each person has his own way of dealing with terror and fear. We need to honor that individual's needs and the fact that our actions can be erratic at times when we are under great stress. Allow for that behavior and know that it can, and will, happen. Above all else, remember that your spouse or partner is afraid of losing you and, like you, needs strength—and space—to heal.

Not only do patients need support, but caretakers also need it to continue to be effective in their role. Venting frustration is crucial for you both. Fortunately, at the same time my support group met, my husband attended a spousal support meeting in another room in the hospital.

In addition, spouses need to have a full life away from the house—a major interest, be it work or a hobby, that allows for necessary distraction and emotional replenishment. My husband always went to the gym to work out before visiting me in the hospital, and on the drive over he listened to Dr. Bernie Siegel's motivation tapes, which he said he found calming.

Ralph also benefited from what he called his parallel support group, a network of intimates available for *him*, in person or by phone, to listen or talk, day or night. These friends also called unfailingly to ask if he was all right, if there was anything *he* needed, or if there was anything they could do for him.

There are many ways you can help your spouse. Encourage him or her to join a support group, get together with friends for dinner, or plan a regular men's or ladies' night. Make arrangements to have someone in the house with you occasionally so your spouse can enjoy the time off with a free mind. This should be an opportunity for him to draw sustenance from friends and from being with other people. It's important he get outside the house to get outside himself.

Major illness isolates you both and it narrows the focus and direction of your life together. Concentrating on healing can be beneficial, but not if that focus is all there is. You need space to breathe, individually, and as a couple.

Ralph and I worked hard to keep our relationship vital and to enhance our time together. We enjoyed renting movies. It broke the tension that was in the house and allowed us to do something fun. He was released from his caretaker role, and we could laugh together. We also ordered take-out dinners at least once a week, which freed him from meal preparation and kitchen cleanup, and gratefully accepted our friends' and neighbors' offers to bring us meals.

We started a weekly date night—an evening set aside just for talking and focused listening. Here is where you as a couple can do some important sharing about how you are each feeling. Lighting a candle and playing music lends a sense of sacredness to these special evenings. Here are some topics for frank but loving conversation:

- What's bothering you most this week?
- What part of my illness is most difficult for you now?

- What aspect of my care is the most unpleasant for you right now?
- If I could do one thing to make life easier for you, what would you like me to do?
- What is your biggest fear or worry right now?
- Which of my behaviors is irritating you most and wish I could change now?
- If there was one friend I could arrange to visit you, whom would you choose?
- What responsibility can I take from you this week to make things easier for you?
- What special thing can we do together to break the tedium (i.e., playing Scrabble, going to a play, or taking a drive in the country)?
- What large goal can we set to reach together (i.e., planning for a weekend getaway)?

While I was recovering I wrote several letters of appreciation to my husband. Writing a few paragraphs saying how much the things your partner is doing mean to you can go a long way toward making his or her burden lighter.

....

An individual doesn't get cancer, a family does.
—TERRY TEMPEST WILLIAMS,
REFUGE

To My Loving Husband

I watched you curl upon the bed tonight
as you lay sleeping
I want you to know that I feel your pain too
I feel your frustration
It gets tough sometimes . . . almost near impossible
We must be strong together
We must be strong for each other
There is madness in God's plan
But know that between my sighs and moans
of desperation
I feel your pain, too.
—MARGIE LEVINE

....

18

Time Balancing

Taking time out for rest and reflection was a necessary part of my recovery. The ringing phones and the steady traffic pattern of hospital staff and well-wishers in and out of my room left me weary. Early on, I became conscious of needing to set time limits with those who came by to see me and with those who called.

I decided to do this after a neighbor appeared in my hospital room carrying a big gift wrapped with a huge bow, and with a nervous smile on her face. I had just gone through major surgery and was still hooked up to IVs with tubes in my nose, chest, and side. Totally exhausted, I prayed for the strength to be able to carry on a conversation. I did my best, but after a time I had to assert myself and ask her to leave so that I could take a nap. Her visit, as well as her gracious departure, were both caring gestures. I was glad to see her, but just didn't have the energy for a long exchange.

Most people, no matter how well-meaning, do not understand the enormous physical and emotional drain one experiences after surgery. Nor did I want to offend anyone. Having company was joyful and healing and certainly boosted my immune system, but a long visit that left me tired and exhausted also undid much of the good receiving company promotes.

So like learning to say "no," I learned to tell my visitors what I needed. When friends called I explained that I'd love for them to come by, but usually set limits on the duration of their stay. I'd even suggest the best times for them to come by; and though it felt awkward to be so assertive, I also learned to tell them when I felt tired or if they had stayed too long. In as gentle and as friendly a way as I could, I'd let them know I'd love them to come back, but right now I was feeling tired and needed a nap. My directness and honesty were appreciated by most friends and helped me recover faster. The support of friends is crucial, but learning to set limits so I was not worn out was an important lesson I took away from my recovery.

19

Journaling

I have kept a personal journal every year since I was eleven years old. These precious books have carried me through many seasons of my life, giving shape to all I experienced.

During my battle for survival, journaling became even more meaningful. I wrote ferociously, describing my fear, frustration, and struggles. I talked about how my back and chest were sore from radiation and how I couldn't wear a bra. I wrote how I couldn't walk into the hospital without getting queasy at the door and about trying to keep up a brave front for my mother. When the weight of illness seemed almost too great to bear, my journal was like a dear friend, available any time day or night, a friend who would not turn away no matter how blue or downhearted I became.

Here in the privacy of a leather-bound book, I could be raw and candid. There was no holding back. I could examine my complex emotions; I could grieve for the old life I wanted to be living; I could find refuge from the consuming pain, nausea, and fear, and it was here where I found courage to raise my sails again. Journaling not only gave me an important outlet for venting feelings safely, it also generated important insights that enhanced my healing. Below are a few lines from my journal:

I couldn't sleep tonight. The hospital was noisy with patients moaning with pain, then this wonderful nurse named Penny came in to ask if I wanted a sleeping pill and we started to talk. She told me her life story and how she got interested in medicine . . . and for a while I forgot I was lying in a hospital bed wrapped in surgical bandages. I think I made a new friend. 12/21/89

NONE of this should happen to a human being!!!! 3/3/90

Today is my second chemo treatment. I came to the hospital for my three-day stay. As I walked into my room I caught my reflection in the mirror and thought this isn't me, this can't be me, this can't really be happening. This is the hardest thing I have ever done. I don't want to be here!!! Be strong, Margie, I keep telling myself, so I don't run out the door. 4/20/90

I want to scream and get it all out!!! The anger, the frustration and this fear. This has got to end soon. It has got to get easier! 8/8/90

Today I went to the beach and sat on the wood rail. It was so peaceful. For a moment I felt alive again. I sat there so taken by the glory of the beauty around me. There was no one there today but I noticed a man with tattered pants meandering toward me with a wobbly gait. As he got closer he walked faster until he came right over to me. I looked up and as if he was talking to an old buddy, he muttered, "There ain't nothing more my friend than this. This is all there is, ya know." Then he smiled and walked away. It was magical. If only this moment could go on forever. 4/2/91

Holding in rage creates negative side effects and eventually the body will be called upon to pay attention. Realizing this encouraged me to write even more, and in fact, new studies show that writing about deeply stressful situations can actually stimulate the immune response and make us feel better. According to one report published in the *Journal of the American Medical Association*, groups of patients randomly assigned to keep journals about their illnesses and how it affected them showed significant symptom reduction over patient groups writing about emotionally neutral topics. Just how the act of writing promotes healing is unclear, although researchers believe that putting our thoughts down on paper is literally *that*: we are *releasing* stress emotionally and toxins physically from our bodies while we simultaneously achieve the inner calm that accompanies self-understanding.

It is only by expressing all that is inside us that purer and purer streams flow forth. Take time in your day to find nourishment by writing about your feelings. Begin by choosing an appealing book with a cover or binding that will draw you to it. You may even want to tuck dried flowers or a photo inside.

Before I start to write, I allow myself a few moments of stillness to gather my thoughts. To get into the journaling habit, try to write in the same place at the same time each day, even for just a few moments and a few quick lines. Very soon journaling will become a special time and anticipated ritual. Be candid and write freely from your heart, expressing your innermost feelings. I date the entries so I can look back later to see how far I have come.

Remember also that like meditation, there is no "right" way to journal. Some people prefer to use a journal as a diary, a daily record of their routines and activities, while others choose to draw rather than write. What matters is using it to honor the way you feel on that particular day. Giving expression to what it feels like to be *you* in that moment in time can be an enriching survival tool.

Journaling can be a powerful way of working through the "big questions" that inevitably push their way into our consciousness when we are fighting for our lives. In his book *Cancer as a Turning Point*, Dr. Lawrence LeShan gives a list of topics for readers to think about. Any of these could also be rich sources for reflection and private commentary. Here is a sampling.

- What is the best thing that ever happened to you? What is the worst?
- If you were asked by a child you love to tell him or her the most important thing that you have learned in your life, what would you reply?
- In each symphony there is a central theme. It has many variations, which appear in different [movements], but underlying them all is the theme. What has been the theme of your life?
- If you could change one decision of your life, what would that be? Why did you make it the way you did? What does this tell you about how you saw yourself and the world at that time? Can you forgive yourself for making that decision the way you did?

- As you look back at your life, what were the moments when you were most yourself? What helped you to do this? What moments were you least yourself? Why do you think this was so?
- During this time, what is the longest time of day for you? What do you mostly feel and think during this time?
- All our lives we try to accomplish something, to do something. What is it that you were trying to do in recent years? Is it still so important to you? How can you finish the attempt so that it ends with harmony and honesty?

People who keep journals have life twice.
—JESSAMYN WEST,
TO SEE THE DREAM

But it's morning. I have been given another day. Another day to hear and read and smell and walk and love and glory.

I am alive for another day.
I think of those who aren't.
—HUGH PRATHER,
NOTES TO MYSELF

First and foremost [writing] reminds us that we are alive
and that it is a gift and a privilege, not a right. Secondly,
writing is survival . . . You must stay drunk on writing
so reality cannot destroy you.
—RAY BRADBURY,
ZEN IN THE ART OF WRITING

20

Nature

When we are going through a crisis we tend to gravitate to a place of comfort, a place that makes us feel safe, that centers and enhances our ability to cope. For me, that place is nature. Spending time in a peaceful outdoor setting became crucial for my healing.

Nature's remarkable healing powers have been acknowledged throughout the ages. The ancients flocked to sacred springs and mountains; the Greeks and Egyptians constructed labyrinthine paths for walking meditations, and the Persians created paradise gardens of streams and fruit trees. Cloistered gardens with flowering trees and fountains gave comfort to the sick during the Middle Ages, while in later times, the tubercular sought relief in the cool mountain air of the Alps and Adirondacks.

There was a time when hospitals, often former monasteries, paid attention to the restorative benefits offered by shaded courtyards and sweeping window views of the surrounding countryside. But that has disappeared as machines, state-of-the-art operating suites, and specialized care units with their functional, fluorescent-lighted spaces have replaced nature with the technology that cures.

Spending so much time confined in hospital rooms with relentless pain, countless needle jabs, and endless nausea made me aware of how much I needed to be outdoors taking in fresh air. Allowing time to be in the midst of nature calmed and quieted me.

After each MRI, CAT scan, blood test, doctor appointment, and medical treatment, I scheduled a pleasurable outing that same day. Not only have I always loved being close to nature, but I have an insatiable passion for the sea. Now the exquisiteness of the dunes and pounding surf had a deeper impact. My husband and I picnicked on every coastal beach along the Boston shoreline. Before each hospital visit, we would map out the special destination for that day. Anticipating the outing enabled me to face the ordeal ahead. The knowledge that there was a reward and a balm in store temporarily ameliorated the grimness of what I faced. And if it rained the day of an appointment, we simply picked a restaurant with an ocean view.

When my surgeries and chemotherapy treatments were

over I began a course of twenty-five radiation sessions. In addition to the sign-up list my women's group had organized for volunteer drivers, other friends phoned to book a day on their own.

Each morning I'd pack a blanket, a thermos of spring water, and a picnic lunch for two. Each of my beloved chauffeurs was faithfully dragged to a sandy beach, pond or reservoir, park, or botanical garden. Along with sharing good food, conversation, and friendship, I always took a few moments to sit in silence. I would bear witness to the natural grace of my surroundings, then connect to my deepest self.

These moments of contemplation and companionship were also punctuated by laughter, joy, and deep appreciation. One January day a friend picked me up from home, coincidentally wearing the same hooded purple parka trimmed with gray fur that I wore. We drove to a sunny Cape Cod beach. There we climbed an icy snowbank, and set up our lounge chairs and our lunch under the deep blue sky as two seagulls watched us from the shore. It was so cold we could see our breath. After all that time in dreary hospital rooms and confined spaces, it was truly a holy moment.

I remember the radiation technician questioning me one morning as I lay prone under the giant machine. Why did I wear a bathing suit under my hospital gown each day?

"I go swimming after I leave here," I responded, thinking nothing of it. Amused, she replied, "Hmm . . . most people leave the hospital and go home to rest!"

It wasn't that I was not tired, but my soul needed nourishment too. Studies show that nature is good medicine. Dr. Roger Ulrich of Texas A&M University found that surgical patients who could view trees and sky recovered faster than patients viewing only four walls. Other studies correlated reductions in pain and stress symptoms to patients who viewed photographs and videotapes of natural scenes.

Swimming that day, and every day I could, under an open sky, with the shadblow and beach roses nearby gently waving to me as ocean breezes rippled past, gave me hope. Being immersed in and buoyed by water helped alleviate my fear. Nature balanced me, and was a continuous stimulant in my healing.

··

I go to nature to be soothed and healed
and to have my senses put in
tune once more.
—JOHN BURROUGHS,
TIME AND CHANGE

Allow me to walk in a meadow
with sunshine and blue sky
and I will confess to being the happiest
woman alive.
—MARGIE LEVINE

The days pass
and from my window
I watch the fullness of the yellow maple tree
slowly losing its brilliance.
The leaves float downward
The sun warms my being
I feel a sudden exuberance . . . a tingling inside
I begin to plan my life recuperated
And I want
to be able to live again.

—MARGIE LEVINE

21

Spiritual Connection

Often, when I am in conversation with a newly diagnosed cancer patient, I will ask whether he or she feels a spiritual connection in his or her life. When the person hesitates it prompts my retort: if you don't know now, you probably will soon.

Severe crisis, along with my increasing emotional vulnerability, heightened my consciousness both of myself and the world around me. In preparing to die, I became cognizant of the unimportance of material possessions. My vision of our purpose on earth, that of giving and receiving love, became more compelling.

I had long felt that something greater than ourselves exists out there, a divine source or divine energy, an essence that touches us and connects us to the physical and intangible aspects of our reality.

Synchronicity is the direct expression of a strong universal force that raises our level of consciousness. It is a way of looking at coincidences as more than just random events. It is an idea embedded in what the theologian Abraham Joshua Heschel calls the concept of "radical amazement."

A series of extraordinary incidents that occurred after my mother's death intensified my understanding of life. Some years later, my husband and I were visiting her grave in upstate New York on our way up north for a weekend in Vermont. As we stood at the cemetery sprinkling white petals over her gravesite from flowers we had taken from her garden and perpetuated in ours, we told her we loved and missed her and felt her energy around us. Afterward, we drove on and checked into a hotel for the night, where we settled into bed and prepared to read. But for the next ninety minutes my bedside light kept flickering on and off, just as it had the day after her death and several times since. We started to smile and I said, "Okay, Celia" (as I liked to call her when she was in a mischievous mood), "we know you're in the room, now knock it off." But I never did read that night.

The following day we arrived in Vermont. We drove well past nightfall over dark, rain-slicked mountain roads trying to find Penelope's, the restaurant we had been told would be the only one open in the area. Ralph was hungry and getting cranky. It seemed as though we had been driving forever up and down country roads, hardly seeing another vehicle. Suddenly, a car swung out of a side road, nearly cutting us off. My husband slammed on the brakes. We followed that car for at least a mile when my husband turned to me and said, "Margie! Look at that license plate!" I peered over the dashboard and read "Celia."

We continued on behind the car for another few miles before it pulled off the road and parked in front of a Laundromat, right next to the restaurant we'd been looking for! Three days later I returned home. That whole month I had been looking for a helper to work with me in closing down our beach house for the season. As I opened my front door, suitcase in hand, I was greeted by a voice coming from my answering machine. "Margie, I found someone for you!" said my neighbor. "She'll be there Monday. She lives close by and her name is . . . Celia."

The memory of these experiences has been a source of strength to me. The unexpected series of synchronistic events after my mother's passing confirmed for me that we are all spiritually connected to one another, here in this life and after. There is a comfort in knowing there is an energy that exists that bridges the physical world around us and the spirit world beyond us. Sensing this in my own situation helped alleviate some of my inner fears.

As my recovery progressed, my understanding of this "interconnectedness" grew deeper. I am aware, as the writer Henrietta Szold said, that "In the light of the spirit there is no ending that is not a beginning."

My thought process has been dramatically reshaped. I now feel a profound sense of inner peace. This fresh perspective is difficult to articulate, but I am aware it all came about during my overwhelming ordeal as I prepared to die.

....

Coincidence is God's way of remaining anonymous.
—UNKNOWN

Spirituality leaps where science cannot yet follow, because science must always test and measure, and much of reality and human experience is immeasurable.
—STARHAWK,
THE SPIRAL DANCE

The voyage of discovery lies not in new vistas but in receiving new eyes.
—RACHEL NAOMI REMEN,
KITCHEN TABLE WISDOM

Perhaps the only limits to the human mind are those we believe in.
—WILLIS HARMAN, FORMER PRESIDENT,
INSTITUTE OF NOETIC *SCIENCES*

Grant that I may not so much seek as to be consoled.
To be understood as to understand
To be loved as to love

For it is in giving that we receive
It is in pardoning that we are pardoned.
And it is in dying that we are born to eternal life.
—ST. FRANCIS PRAYER

Every action in our lives touches some chord
That vibrates in eternity
when we spend our time very well
the reverberation is also very beautiful.
—GURUMAYI CHIDVILASANANDA,
RESONATE WITH STILLNESS

22

Prayer

For thousands of years, in countries around the world, the faithful have looked to divine intervention to relieve pain and suffering and impart healing. Religion, too, has played a role in medicine for centuries. The first hospitals were operated by monks and the religious orders have always cared for the sick. But with advances in medical science— bringing antibiotics and other modern "miracles"—the medical community no longer needed to call on God's healing.

Today, our thinking is shifting and once again there is

wide acknowledgment of the power of prayer. More than half of U.S. medical schools, including Harvard, Duke, and Johns Hopkins, teach courses on issues involving spirituality and prayer. What was once considered only anecdotal evidence that a belief in an all-powerful divine source has a positive effect on healing is now being supported by a wide range of clinical research. Dr. Larry Dossey, a former internist and a best-selling author, has been a major force in promoting the effectiveness of prayer among the medical establishment. In study after study, Dossey found that "Faith empowers science. If you join reason with faith, then you have something more powerful than either."

The research suggests that prayer plays a vital role in healing. Although it does not always cure, it promotes spiritual well-being and reduces anxiety and depression. Prayer may be effective regardless of religious affiliation, how, or where it is performed, or who actually performs it. Some studies indicate that *prayerfulness*—the act where one surrenders to the great mystery and aligns oneself with the will of God—may be even more beneficial than asking for a specific outcome.

These studies—more than 250 according to the National Institutes of Health—are creating a picture of a highly connected and interactive universe. Two studies I find most intriguing concern intercessory prayer—praying for someone at a distance.

In a landmark 1996 double-blind study led by Dr. Elisabeth Targ, twenty patients with advanced AIDS received healing prayers over a concentrated period while twenty other patients did not. In order to control for the power of suggestion, the healers worked at a distance receiving the barest of personal information about the patient each would be praying for—name, lab reports, and a picture. Neither the patients nor the doctors knew who was receiving prayers. After six months, the researchers found that the prayer recipients had notable differences from the control group, including significantly fewer doctor visits and hospital stays. Still another study enlisted Buddhist monks in Tibet, who prayed for patients at the very hour during which their physicians were performing surgery. Postoperative complications were found to be reduced by half—another compelling result that would confirm how one person can, merely by intention, influence the physical well-being of another.

"To be healed," writes Dr. Lewis Mehl-Madrona in his book *Coyote Medicine*, "we need to believe in the possibility of healing and in a greater world, and in higher powers than our own. We must be willing to use anything that works, regardless of our theoretical positions. *Because if it works, it's good medicine*."

I not only personally prayed to a higher being but also welcomed prayer offers from kindly visitors. Sometimes, I humbly requested it. I encouraged friends to put my name on prayer lists and healing circles. I believe that if one prayer can help, many can help that much more.

While vacationing for the first time after completing treatment, I was staying in a motel with Ralph in Boca Raton, Florida. One morning as I was resting on the couch the maid arrived to straighten up. As she dusted we chatted, and when she learned of my horrific plight, she insisted I return to my suite during her lunch break at noon.

Sure enough, with crumpled sandwich bags in hand, the maid and three energetic cohorts appeared to offer blessings. Standing over me as I lay across the sagging couch, with bowed heads and joined hands, they began chanting to the gods. In unison and a foreign tongue, the four Cuban ladies bellowed out their prayers and praised the Lord. With swaying hips and sweating brows, the maids pleaded for my miraculous recovery. As I heard them sing together in perfect harmony, chills traveled up my spine. I was touched by the profound caring of these four strangers.

Healing comes in many packages. For some, prayer is the steering wheel, for others, it's the spare tire, Corrie ten Boom observed wryly in *Don't Wrestle, Just Nestle*. In my life, prayer is a great and various garden but in particular, it is a channel for concentrating positive thoughts and practicing what George Leonard and Michael Murphy describe as "Focused Surrender."

Focused Surrender is seen by many as the pivotal piece that precedes God's grace—that which seems miraculous. It was at just such a moment, following a period of concentrated mental effort, that a young researcher at Stanford Research Institute, succeeded in coaxing movement from a huge and sensitive magnetometer by his will alone. Over and over again the man tried to stimulate a response but to no avail until, exhausted and frustrated, he gave up. Suddenly, in that instant, the needle jumped! Along with others, the researcher repeated these efforts many times, and later spoke of using his will to effect a connection with the instrument, which would then "coalesce . . . into a field of palpable energy. I'd feel myself coming into the magnetic field and pulsing it to respond," he stated. "Then when there would be a moment of total surrender, the response would occur." In other words, embedded somewhere in the tango of effort and intent, resting and yielding, is the place where miracles can occur.

The young man's story greatly reinforced my use of "surrender." By drawing consciousness and intentionality—the force of my desire to get well—together with prayer, I believed that the very act of holding my hands together closed a field of healing energy around me. But in asking for grace, for God's divine rhythm to reveal itself, I also allowed myself to surrender to it.

God always hears our prayers, author and spiritualist Rosemary Ellen Guiley tells us, and answers them in one of three ways: *This; not this; not yet.* I was doing all I humanly could—but I instinctively knew the final piece was to *let go*—and then let God respond.

Through my prayerful expression, I fell into a divine dialogue that brought luminous and healing light into my everyday living.

Create a Synchronized Prayer Chain

Having directed prayer sent your way from caring friends and family can be a boost to the healing process. Ask at least five people you know to be part of a prayer chain that sends you healing energy at a specified time of each day. The energy can be in a thought form picturing you healed and well, it may be in the form of ritualized prayer with your name mentioned, or it may just be a few words asking the Divine for improvement for your highest good. Ask each of these friends to ask more friends, so that the benefit of the focused energy you receive is even more intensified. At the appointed hour (be sure to adjust it to various time zones, if necessary), take a moment to absorb those energized thoughts and open your palms briefly to create a channel for the healing being sent to you.

The prayer chain can be a wonderful project for a friend who wants to be of help but does not know what to do. Through creative networking, dozens upon dozens of prayers may cross vast oceans in the service of your healing. Use e-mail to make your request to send prayers, along with instructions of how to begin, or you can arrange that a brief announcement be made at your place of worship.

Not only does a prayer chain offer support for the person in need, but it also lets those caring others feel they are a vital part of your healing experience.

Another path to consider is a formal service known as Silent Unity, a more than century-old prayer ministry, offering prayer twenty-four hours a day throughout the world to people of *all* faiths. I use it both for myself and others regularly. Each phoned-in name is put on an official prayer list for thirty days. Hundreds of devoted volunteers pray daily for the person in need. At the end of the thirty days, one may phone the name in again. Donations are not mandatory but appreciated. The Unity Hotline may be reached by phone (816) 969-2000, by fax (816) 251-3554 or on the web (*www.unityworldhq.org*).

Also excellent and providing twenty-four-hour service is the World Ministry of Prayer ([800] 421-9600). You can also go to www.postaprayer.com, which accepts prayer requests. I am glad to spread the word of such good works.

What you see with your eyes shut is what matters.

—LOME DEER,

SIOUX MEDICINE MAN

I surrender to the natural rhythm of life. I will put forth
my best effort, summon all my strength, and then allow
the perfection of God's plan to reveal itself.

—MARGIE LEVINE

23

Local Clergy

I was receptive when a relative asked if she could send her chaplain to my home. It was comforting having him as a receptive listener. I appreciated the depth of his caring and the blessing he offered me.

I always had many meaningful sessions with the hospital clergy on staff when I was an inpatient. Whenever I returned to the hospital for tests or chemo (and I did, often), the first day or two were especially lonely. There were many strange faces—nurses and technicians I didn't know, and new doctors—all of them coming through to poke and prod. When night settles on a hospital floor, long after the tests are done and your visitors have gone home, after the last shift has changed and you are alone with your fear, the silence can be oppressive. I craved a feeling of connection to someone who could be a guide and support.

So I always made it a point of phoning for the hospital clergy. Most hospitals provide twenty-four-hour on-call service. I never knew who would appear—a priest, a minister, or a rabbi. It didn't matter. Their religious affiliation had no bearing on the offered gift, for it was truly compassion that was the key. They helped soften the transition of moving from home to hospital; were always receptive to hearing my fears, never judging or proselytizing. They offered me such healing warmth and comfort that it became a ritual for me to call upon them whenever I was to stay longer than overnight.

24

Nourishment

During my cancer treatment my oncologist informed me of the foods I'd be most able to tolerate. I also read nutrition booklets from the American Cancer Society and went over various programs with hospital dieticians who visited me in my room.

I was aware of the need to take in an adequate amount of protein and about trying to get down something that was nourishing. Chemotherapy can leave the mouth with a metallic taste. You may also experience a temporary adverse reaction to some familiar foods. It is important to eat what pleases you during this time of healing and to listen to what your body is telling you.

Poached eggs (well done) and whole wheat toast were easy to tolerate and became a staple. When I added to that a serving of chickpeas I easily fulfilled my daily protein requirement. My oncologist also encouraged me to include fish and chicken in my diet for nutritional support and to eat some red meat to replenish the B vitamins lost through chemotherapy. I incorporated all meat into my diet very sparingly, because chicken and beef are each injected with hormones and antibiotics (which is particularly problematic for people with hormone receptor type cancer such as breast cancer). Because I did not feel comfortable eating a lot of meat, when I did I tried to make sure it was organic or wild (like venison) and thoroughly cooked. Studies indicate that up to one third of all meat products carry E coli bacteria. Because I was immuno-suppressed, I didn't want to take unnecessary risks.

Nevertheless I found plenty to eat during treatment. Fruit popsicles, frozen bananas on a stick, frozen grapes, and lollipops were soothing to my throat. Watermelon was easy to digest and tasted wonderful. I enjoyed peaches and mixed berries. Ice cream and banana milk shakes provided nourishment and were delicious and filling at the same time.

Tapioca and rice puddings were two of my favorites. Sometimes I added chopped apples and raisins. Flavored puddings such as butterscotch and vanilla, which I would often top with sliced bananas or sprinkle with granola, were soft and satisfying. Cans of liquid Ensure supplied nutrients on days when food was not appealing.

I forced myself to drink as much bottled water and flavored seltzer as I could to flush out body toxins. After I completed a chemotherapy session I drank ginger tea and found it helped with the lingering nausea. Before you try it, be sure to consult your doctor first. While the nausea-fighting properties of ginger are excellent, ginger can also inhibit blood-clotting and in rare instances trigger gastrointestinal bleeding. If you are undergoing chemotherapy and your platelet levels are below sixty thousand (the number that indicates compromised clotting ability) adding ginger can create more complications. On the other hand, ginger ale poses no such difficulties. Most carbonated beverages use artificial flavoring or contain tiny amounts of ginger.

Another tea I was able to tolerate was green tea. In fact, green tea contains large amounts of polyphenols, natural substances that act as antioxidants and may thereby help prevent the cell changes that cause cancer. Black tea is also an excellent source of polyphenols, while herbal tea contains none at all. Recent studies published in the *Journal of the National Cancer Institute* suggest that the polyphenol EGCG found in green tea selectively destroys cancerous cells while leaving healthy cells unharmed, and may therefore offer a promising new avenue for treatment.

My recovery owed much to the array of healthy foods I was able to consume. Eating well lifted my spirits and enhanced my state of well-being during those months of treatment.

25

Veggie Overdosing

A few months after my medical protocol was behind me, my appetite improved. I once again started to crave regular meals.

Having always had an interest in healthy eating, I now began to hone in on newly published data on nutrition and disease. I was encouraged by the research linking low fat–high fiber diets to a lowered risk of fifteen types of cancer, including cancers of the colon, breast, and lung. This "new anti-cancer diet," as Dr. Andrew Weil describes it, provides rich troves of natural antioxidants that protect cells from damage caused by cancer-causing agents.

Fiber is like a broom to our digestive system, sweeping waste from the stomach to the bowel and thus reducing the length of time toxic substances stay inside us. Biologist and cancer researcher Dr. Jonathan Yavelow explains the enormous boost fiber gives our immune systems when we eat five to nine servings each day of fruits, vegetables, and beans or legumes:

> Legumes have a molecule in them that survives cooking and digestion. It remains active in the intestine blocking the conversion of normal cells into cancer cells. Proteases are enzymes that can increase tumor cells ability to grow. People who eat a lot of legumes tend to have a higher rate of protease inhibitors in their diets and experience a lower risk of various types of cancer.

Because food plays such a vital role in our state of wellness, eating consciously was *one* way I could be in charge of what happened to me. I decided to follow the diet the studies indicated most effectively discourages the growth of cancer, or its return. What I do is quite simple: I overdose on veggies!

Fruits and vegetables are my mainstay. Among the quantities of fresh vegetables I eat are carotenoid-rich carrots, yams, squash, pumpkin, and turnips, which have been found to be effective immune system stimulants. Dark leafy vegetables like romaine lettuce, arugula, collard greens, and kale are particularly helpful in detoxifying the liver. This is especially important since that organ is carrying an overload from both the disease and the toxic therapy if chemo is being used.

Research studies show that large intakes of broccoli in particular can help prevent lung cancer. Whereas I read that the average American eats seven pounds of broccoli a year, I eat seven pounds each *week*. Broccoli is a cruciferous vegetable, part of the Brassica family, that includes cabbage, kale, cauliflower, and brussels sprouts. Even in ancient times, the power of these greens was recognized. The Roman poet Cato wrote, "The cabbage surpasses all other vegetables." Cruciferous vegetables contain vitamin C and folic acid (an important B vitamin) as well as beta carotene, potassium, and vitamin K. Most important is its wealth of sulfuraphane, which stimulates the production of enzymes found to defuse and expel potential carcinogens from our bodies.

Of all the vegetables that contain sulfuraphane, broccoli is the queen. In fact, researchers believe that intestinal bacteria act on broccoli to produce even more sulfuraphane. This substance is regarded as such a potential effective cancer fighter, researchers are experimenting with it and testing its benefits for use in other forms of cancer treatment.

And because I also consume enormous bowls of salads of all types, I make sure to have an abundance of fresh lettuces, cabbage, onions, garlic, and fresh ginger in my home at all times (ginger contains twelve antioxidants and can be kept in the freezer for months if well wrapped).

Eating healthfully is one of the easiest and most enjoyable things you can do for your well-being. You will notice you feel better once you start eliminating high-fat foods and eating all the fruits and vegetables you want.

Sharing the Ritual

As soon as my appetite returned I began a weekly ritual I follow faithfully today.

My Monday morning preparation begins with soaking, scrubbing, cutting, steaming, and bagging a variety of vegetables to enhance my health. (I always use vinegar, a natural cleansing agent, when I wash vegetables, even if the label states "prewashed," as an extra precaution against pesticide residue.) After I have washed and scrubbed my weekly staple of fresh vegetables, I put one-quarter aside for later use.

In a large pot on my stove I steam a combination of many vegetables using the smallest amount of water possible, as some vitamins and beneficial plant compounds leach out into the cooking water. (Note: It has been found that steaming vegetables for three to five minutes releases more nutrients than eating them raw.) For variety I add four additional vegetables each week to my regular carrot and broccoli mix. These may include zucchini, turnips, tomatoes, cabbage, kale, eggplant, beets, cauliflower, butternut squash, red, yellow, and green peppers, spinach, corn, collard greens, parsnips, green peas, shiitake mushrooms, yams, or celery. (Button mushrooms, peanuts, and celery have been identified as natural carcinogens when eaten in excess. When consumed in moderation, there is no harm.) Be mindful of cooking time, as overcooking can destroy crucial nutrients. Drain the vegetables while they are still al dente and retain the cooking water.

During the last minutes of steaming I add a container of firm, low-fat tofu to the steam pot for protein. (On occasion I will add pieces of fish or free-range chicken breasts that I have separately prepared.) To concentrate the flavor, I sometimes steam the tofu separately for two minutes with onions and garlic, a hunk of fresh ginger, two tablespoons of tamari sauce, and a squeeze of fresh lemon, then add the mixture to the vegetable pot.

When the steaming is complete, drain and retain the water. I drink the steaming water as a hot tea. It is rich in vitamins and makes a healthy broth.

In another pot I prepare a package of either whole wheat pasta, brown rice, couscous, quinoa, pearl barley, legumes, or some other carbohydrate rich in fiber. When ready, I drain and combine with the vegetables.

When the vegetable pot cools to room temperature, I divide the nutritious potpourri into five glass bowls for weekday meals and refrigerate. (If you use Tupperware, wait until the mixture cools before you fill the containers, and to reheat, transfer to glass. If using plastic wrap when reheating, don't let it directly touch the food, for heated plastic releases toxic chemicals suspected of causing cancer.)

My cooked vegetables done, I now return to the remaining cut vegetables set aside earlier. I keep these raw and bag them in Ziploc bags. Sliced carrots, cucumbers, zucchini, and peppers make great snacks. I eat them with a touch of onion salt, garlic powder, or garlic spray.

I vary the routine according to the season. During the

summer, I slice and wrap cantaloupe, kiwi, mango, straw-berries, grapes, and blueberries. Frozen grapes and bananas on a popsicle stick are satisfying snacks on hot days. In the fall and winter, I will steam apples, pears, parsnips, yams, turnips, prunes, figs, and raisins; and I keep oranges and bananas in my home all year. I also rely on fresh herbs such as basil, oregano, caraway seed, nutmeg, clove, and all-spice. These natural seasonings vary my preparations and awaken the flavors—and all of them have been found to have antioxidant activity.

My Monday morning event has become a sacred ritual in my life. I have fun creating new vegetable combinations and have found Deborah Madison's *Vegetarian Cooking for Everyone* an inspiring addition to my kitchen library. And when I eat salads, I enjoy experimenting with ingredients and dressings. I like to include citrus fruits (preferably organic because of their skin) such as oranges, grapefruit, tangerines, lemons, and limes, all recognized as possessing anticancer activity. And because citrus skin is also thought to contain the cancer-fighting substance D-limonene, I let it do double duty in tea (which I make by boiling the skin) and in salad dressings, where adding a teaspoon of zest intensifies the flavor wonderfully.

In your quest to be inventive try surfing the web for ideas. The food magazines all have websites featuring recipes, and epicurious.com is another excellent resource to help expand your vegetable repertoire.

Aside from building up my immune system, I truly enjoy healthy eating. I make an effort to limit my intake of refined sugar, saturated fat, and processed foods. Reading labels has become a natural part of my routine. Food and drug laws require the most dominant ingredient in a product be labeled first, so when the word "sugar" appears first on a cereal box, I know the product is one I want to avoid. I look instead for grain products that list 100 percent whole wheat as the first ingredient, and I try to stay away from anything with added Karo or corn syrup and limit my intake of foods with hydrogenated oil (especially prevalent in crackers, cookies, and most processed baked goods).

I try to buy organic products when possible. Because my system is less resilient than it was after having been immuno-suppressed, I have not resumed eating raw fish of any kind. Sushi can carry parasites and raw clams a certain form of hepatitis. I used to love to sit on our deck and enjoy a glass of wine and a tray of clams on the half shell with my husband as the sun set. We still have the wine at sunset, but don't take unnecessary chances. Instead I've found healthier substitutes like cooked shrimp with cocktail sauce and a vegetable platter with hummus. Watching the sky break into flames of vibrant color seems just as exhilarating.

In recent years I have discovered tofu (made from soybeans). Stir-fried or steamed, as in Asian cooking, it is a delicious and versatile alternative to animal protein. The isoflavones in soy foods such as tofu, tempeh, and soymilk appear to be highly beneficial. These foods also contain a compound called *genistein*, which inhibits the growth of blood vessels near tumors, necessary for their survival. (Note that highly processed forms of soy such as Asian soy sauce, soy oil, and soy "burgers" may not have these natural cancer protection compounds in the concentration that soybeans and fresh tofu offer.) (Refer to the bibliography for info on this.)

I include high-fiber foods like beans (red, navy, kidney, lima, lentils, etc.), cereals, bran and wheat germ, whole wheat grain breads, pastas, and rice in my diet every day, and for snacks I nibble on dried apricots, figs, and air-popped popcorn.

On weekends I am flexible with food choices. I'll eat red meat on occasion and at summer barbecues I will never pass up a hot dog on a grill. Sometimes I feel restraining oneself in social situations can create such discomfort and isolation that the negative hormones associated with that are more harmful than just indulging for the moment. The robust pleasure derived from an occasional treat translates into a form of healing, too. Eat well but think moderation!

Celebration Stew

(SERVES 8)

A special annual ritual that I share with a Cape Cod neighbor is an autumn harvest celebration, where we prepare a fancy vegetable stew. We begin by saying a brief meditative prayer outside. We open our palms and give gratitude to the earth's bounty and to our friendship. Then, with fire blazing, classical music in the background, and a bottle of chilled wine, we chop, cut, and cook all day. By evening's end, after we have sampled bowls of our warmed brew, we label and freeze the finished product. This preparation provides us both with lots of hearty meals for cold winter nights. Not only is the concoction delicious, but each precious container is full of TLC—the best medicine of all.

Six 12-ounce cans chicken or vegetable broth
Two 36-ounce cans stewed tomatoes
2 cups water
Two 6-ounce cans tomato paste
4 onions, chopped
2 large bunches spinach, chopped
1 bunch parsley, chopped
1 clove garlic, chopped
1 bunch carrots, scraped and sliced
4–6 parsnips, scraped and sliced
2 turnips, sliced thin
2 cups green beans, ends trimmed
1 bunch collard greens, chopped
2 zucchini, sliced
1 small head cabbage, chopped
1 cup barley
1 cup lentils

1 cup dried yellow peas
1 handful fresh basil, chopped
Salt and pepper to taste

Place all ingredients into a 12-quart pot. Bring to a boil and simmer for 1 hour. Serve with salad and fresh crusty bread. *Bon appétit!*

....

Food is medicine and medicine
is food.
—HIPPOCRATES

Five Vital Cancer Fighting Foods

Oranges—High in fiber, vitamin C, and the antioxidant flavonoid. Studies show the best way to prevent cell damage is to increase your consumption of antioxidants.

Cooked Tomatoes—Lycopene is the substance that gives tomatoes their vibrant color. It is also a powerful antioxidant that may lower the risk of prostate, colon, and cervical cancer. It is absorbed best when taken with olive oil (as in pasta sauce).

Fish—Salmon, mackerel, and herring are rich in omega-3 fatty acids that appear to yield small but significant preventative effects in certain cancers. Other good omega-3 sources are found in canola oil and walnuts.

Garlic—The most pungent member of the onion family and valued for its medicinal benefits, garlic can aid in blood detoxification during chemo or radiation. Best eaten raw.

100 Percent Whole Wheat Bread—An immune system booster, studies show whole wheat can help protect against some forms of cancer and prevent further illness.

According to a recent study published in the newsletter of the Tufts University School of Medicine, the three most nutritious fruits are guava, watermelon, and grapefruit. Those most often loaded with pesticides are strawberries, apples, and cherries. Other studies show that blueberries, blackberries, and raspberries, contain a special antioxidant called *ellagic acid*, believed to prevent cellular changes that can lead to cancer. Berries are very high in vitamin C, which is thought to reduce the risk of cancer and other diseases. (Refer to the bibliography for info on this.)

2 6

Phytochemicals

I take vitamins every day. My physician has encouraged me to include 400 units of vitamin E, 1,200 mg of calcium, and 50 mg of the trace mineral selenium. I also take a multivitamin in a clear gelatin-coated capsule, a form I find preferable to the dye-colored coatings generally used to encapsulate vitamin supplements. In addition, I support my immune system each day by taking a supplement of phytonutrients. The American Cancer Society has recommended taking cancer-fighting phytochemicals as a powerful way to improve health.

The phytonutrient complex I take is a proprietary blend of twelve whole raw fruits and vegetables—broccoli, brussels sprouts, cabbage, carrots, cauliflower, garlic, kale, onions, tomatoes, turnips, papayas, and pineapple—which have been allowed to fully vine-ripen prior to harvesting, then are flash freeze-dried. Allowing fruits and vegetables to fully ripen on the vine maximizes their vitamins, minerals, and newly discovered compounds called phytochemicals. Phytochemicals are the substances responsible in part for giving fruits and vegetables their brilliant colors and special flavors, but also contain important molecules. These molecules have shown evidence of supporting various defense mechanisms in the body, including detoxifying contaminants and inhibiting the growth of cancer cells.

Unless fruits and vegetables are picked at the moment they reach maturity, their distinctive health benefits diminish. Yet most of the produce we buy at the market—even when organically grown and marked "vine-ripened"—has been green-harvested. They have been picked before they are fully vine-ripened, leaving their most valuable nutrients behind in the roots and stems of the plants. This may be why animals rarely forage for tender shoots and roots. Instinctively they know when the nutrients are at their optimum.

The phytonutrient complex comes in capsule or bulk form, tastes like vegetables, and can be added to salads, dips, and vegetable drinks and juices. I enjoy it in the form of a healthy snack that looks and tastes like gummy bears. Each chewy candy contains the same healthful array of whole fruits and vegetables as the powdered phytonutrients. I prefer to save them for a sweet snack at the end of the day.

My nutrition-giving gummy bears are delicious and economical. Although there is no substitute for fresh fruits and vegetables and good eating, phytonutrients offer strong protective benefits. To find out more about phytonutrients and phytochemicals—or to purchase them directly—you can e-mail your request to *phytohealth4 @yahoo.com* or send a stamped self-addressed envelope to Phytohealth 4, P.O. Box 554, Ashland, MA 01721.

27

Energy Healer

The feeling of desperation can motivate one to try almost anything with the hope of finding a cure. I was receptive to blending traditional medicine with alternative treatment and investigated all options.

In my search I found a woman claiming success with the technique of "energy healing." By activating a divine energy source she said she could invigorate my immune systems to promote healing. I decided to give it a try.

Twice a week Channah appeared at my door. Dressed in a long flowing skirt with her hair tightly wrapped under a black silk scarf, she greeted me with tape recorder and music in hand. The ritual was always the same. As I lay on a wooden coffee table, eyes closed, Channah's swirling arms danced wildly above my prone body to pulsating music. Then, while kneeling beside me, she'd utter in a strong voice a series of prolonged, guttural sounds I didn't understand. She recited a series of Hebrew prayers from the Bible and concluded the hour by holding her hands against my forehead. I always felt the heat radiating from her sweaty palms.

Sometimes the sessions felt strange and I wondered what I was really doing. But "all healing is self-healing," as Albert Schweitzer once said. We know, for example, that while an orthopedist can reset a broken bone, it is the body itself that does the actual healing. What the physician has done is to facilitate that innate process. I liked to believe that Channah was doing much the same by realigning my energy flow in order to eliminate blockages and obstacles to self-healing. This is what I told myself, anyway.

Then a remarkable occurrence happened after my doctor informed me I would be unable to tolerate my third scheduled chemotherapy treatment and that I would have to postpone it. He said I was neutropenic, meaning that my white blood count was seriously low, thereby making me highly susceptible to infection. Doctors do not like to administer chemotherapy when a patient is in this state. I was asked to leave the clinic and to go home. This news disappointed and unsettled me. I did not want to prolong my treatments or postpone them; I was desperately anxious to finish the prescribed program and resume a normal life.

The following day Channah arrived at my home for our regular session. For the entire hour we focused only on boosting my blood count. Together we envisioned the white cells increasing.

Five days later I returned to the Dana-Farber Cancer Institute. After having blood drawn, the nurses told me my counts had risen significantly. My body was ready to handle the injections. The staff was surprised by the quick turnaround.

The dramatic change appeared to be a direct result of the energy healing session. Encouraged, I made sure I documented the data. I continued to feel that so long as this, or any other alternate modality I heard about, did no harm, I would look at it proactively, and approach it with an open mind.

The cluster of therapies that are called "energy medicine" is gaining wide popularity as an effective means to control pain and enhance relaxation and healing. While techniques vary, almost all of them use hands-on, non-invasive techniques, and all are based on the principle that human bodies are composed of vibrating fields of energy that become disturbed or blocked with illness. Two of the most popular among energy therapies are Therapeutic Touch and Reiki.

Therapeutic Touch is primarily the province of registered nurses, now said to number more than thirty thousand practicing nationwide in two hundred hospitals. Its name is a misnomer, because proponents believe that energy fields extend out from the body for several inches making actual physical touch unnecessary. Practitioners prepare themselves by assuming a relaxed, tranquil state before beginning to pass their hands a few inches over the patient's body in slow, rhythmic movements like sensors, to identify and eliminate blockages in the patient's energy field to facilitate healing. When a blockage is identified, the nurse healer uses downward sweeping motions, working to "knead" the energy field smooth again. Used as a supplement to standard care, the procedure lasts anywhere from ten to thirty minutes, and concludes as the practitioner's hands are passed over the patient's body again in a final effort at energy transfer. Therapeutic Touch is said to improve postoperative circulation and breathing, and to help surgical wounds and sutures heal faster. Patients report pain relief and increased well-being.

Reiki (pronounced ray-key) is an ancient healing art that translates as "universal life energy." A session takes place with the receiver either sitting or lying down, fully clothed, while the practitioner gently uses his hands to directly conduct healing energy to the chakras (or energy centers) of the body of the person being assisted. Like Therapeutic Touch, one can also practice Reiki on oneself, by placing one's own hands on the part of the body in need of healing. Reiki itself does not heal but is instead an energy transfer from a universal energy field or higher spiritual power that creates a subtle yet powerful transformation. A typical treatment can include either physical touch or nonphysical touch, in which case the energy is moved by the practitioner's hands being placed a few inches above the body. A session can last thirty to sixty minutes and is repeated over a period of days, or even months. During the treatment period, the patient is urged to drink plenty of water to help expel body toxins.

At Columbia Presbyterian Medical Center in New York City, Dr. Mehmet Oz, a cardiac surgeon, has experimented with trained healers in the operating room giving hands-on energy healing as he performs coronary bypass surgery. His research has shown that patients receiving such treatment had faster recoveries than those who did not receive such treatment.

Energy-based therapies appear to be promising complements to traditional medical techniques and postoperative care. In fact, the world's first Touch Research Institute has been founded at the University of Miami Medical School to further explore and document the benefits of Therapeutic Touch. And, of course, it was actually Hippocrates himself who described the healing powers of "the force that flows from many people's hands." I believe we must remain open to the gifts from the universe.

....

But all God's angels come to us disguised.
—JAMES RUSSELL LOWELL

Flowing with the universe,
being a channel for its energy,
not judging another's path,
celebrating this gift of life,
doing only what you love and

taking the risk to do it.
Owning your reality,
knowing life is fleeting
and must be lived now.
—SUSAN HAYWARD,
BAG OF JEWELS

28

Exercise and

Movement

A day after my surgery the medical hospital staff got me up, weary but walking, in order to clear my lungs and prevent pneumonia. Every day thereafter I walked the hospital corridors, dragging my IV pole. When I was discharged and home recovering in bed, movement remained important because in its absence muscle atrophy sets in and the blood does not circulate well. I also did full body stretches in bed, reaching my arms and legs forward and backward, and chair exercises, building up from five to ten to fifteen minutes at a time.

Getting the body mobile again is vital, and is a process that takes time, discipline, and patience. We know that exercise as a rule promotes general well-being; but for cancer patients studies suggest specific benefits regarding mood, sleep, digestion, and a faster recovery of energy levels following chemotherapy and radiation treatments.

When I felt a little stronger I practiced yoga on my bedroom floor. Other forms of nonaerobic exercise, tai chi and qigong, are also ways to enhance one's strength and flexibility, sharpen one's mental focus, and reduce stress. In fact, qigong (pronounced chee-goong)—a traditional Chinese system for attaining balance within one's body and between oneself and the natural world—may be particularly effective. There is increasing evidence that patients who practice its system of moving and breathing exercises, which are interspersed with meditation, have an increased number of "helper" T cells and NK cells, which may enhance the immune system function in patients with cancer. (A new study funded by a $100,000 grant from the Charles A. Dana Foundation is currently comparing qigong's health and immune system benefits with those produced by more traditional exercise programs.)

When I felt better and was able to leave the house I began moderate aerobic exercise. I found that just being outside and walking for even fifteen minutes, taking fresh air into my lungs, elevated my mood and boosted my energy level. It took my mind off the trauma as well as the unrelenting nausea and pain. I always chose a scenic spot for my walks. When friends called, and I was able, I'd suggest driving to a beach to walk near the sand and surf.

Swimming has always been my favorite form of exercise. I would always be the first one to jump into a cool lake, and very often the only one. For years I have had a personal ritual where I mark my calendar with the date of my last swim the previous season and try to beat it. I recall many late Octobers on Cape Cod where I was the only swimmer in the ocean, paddling around a few floating buoys and swarming minnows. Runners and ordinary folks walking the beach wrapped in scarfs and parkas would stop, look askance, and call out, "Chilly in there?" Sometimes it was so cold I could only bob my head "yes." But when I would rush home and feel the steaming heat from my outdoor shower, nothing felt more joyous or life affirming.

In the days just after my final radiation treatment I could see white caps from my sunroom window. I wasn't surprised when the radio warned of high seas and a distant hurricane. I have always found storms in the ocean exhilarating and knew instinctively I needed to be with the surf and waves. We are so fortunate that the beach where we live is relatively calm and without an undertow. So as my husband watched snuggled in the car with the heat blasting, I trekked through the blowing sand to the water's edge, dropped my towel, and plunged in. As I battled the waves curious onlookers awaiting the oncoming storm would stop and point at the spectacle of the crazy lady out there in the surf. The surf was as rough as I had ever seen it, but at that moment I felt strong and alive again as I had not since my cancer diagnosis. I imagined I was washing away my fear and pain and that they were floating out to sea. It was a powerful moment, a turning point.

Any form of prescribed exercise you are able to tolerate can work wonders toward enhancing the goal of wellness. A recent study published in the journal *Cancer* concluded that patients engaging in regular aerobic exercise following their course of chemotherapy recovered their stamina faster than those who rested instead. Be aware that doctors advise patients to wait twenty-four hours after a chemo infusion before exercising, and always remember to check your exercise regimen with your physician.

29

Music and Sound

Music has the power to open our senses, lighten our mood, and give expression to our feelings. Perhaps more than any of the five senses, music does the most to deepen our responses to the world. Its power is immediate. Our bodies respond to sound as sunflowers bend to sunlight. Whether we are stimulated by a dynamic drumbeat or soothed by a soft melody, our bodies synchronize instinctively with what we hear. Like human tuning forks, we drum our fingers, nod our heads; our muscles go slack, our consciousness is transported.

Throughout time man has recognized music's phenomenal power to engage us emotionally. As Dr. Andrew Weil has suggested, try turning down the sound on your TV next time you watch a drama or action-adventure show. Those swelling soundtracks are the trip wires that bring on our tears, make our hearts pound, our palms sweat. Music has the incredible ability to alter the very nature of our emotional experience. The response is instinctive. And so it is with health.

Research now documents the therapeutic role of music and sound on our well-being. The new science of psychoacoustics shows how sound waves that stimulate the ear influence the body. Vibration moves energy and blockages are opened within us, allowing us to be more receptive to healing. Listening to calm, melodic sounds slows our brain waves; the mind and heart cease racing; breathing deepens. Music that is rhythmic is a physiological stimulant that energizes us, adding to our endurance, strength, and motivation.

I grew up in a musical family so it was natural for me to turn to music. My mother was a songwriter who composed ballads and had live recording sessions in our home. At many a holiday celebration the family gathered around the piano to sing. Music and song were strong, positive forces for me—a connection to loved ones and happy memories.

When my mother and I were going through our convalescence together, we had a favorite song by Hall and Oates that became "our song." Whenever we would spend time together we would play it, and always she would get up and dance. After she died, one of the things that I had delivered to me from her home was her precious stereo. Eventually, my husband set it up in our Cape Cod home. As he was working I called from the bedroom to my husband, busy pulling wires together, to hurry, that I felt a message coming from my musical mom. He ignored me, as he usually does when I say such things. When the stereo's radio at last popped on, I was elated to hear my beautiful living room enveloped with song. And then I came into the room, touched the dial—and instantaneously, the Hall and Oates tune filled the room. The energy charged my soul. I was awestruck by the synchronistic moment.

I was encouraged to use music to stimulate my body's potential to heal. I drew eclectically on classical, folk, and contemporary favorites for a relaxation tape to use as I prepared for surgery, chemo treatments, medical appointments, and in moments when I needed to quiet my fear and uncertainty. Often while listening to music I practiced my visualized imagery. As I recovered, I varied my music choices according to my mood. I put together a tape of favorites—personal "anthems" I could depend on to lighten my mood when I was blue and energize my fighting spirit. My tape player was my constant companion. Friends shared their favorite music with me. And when I felt better I went to as many outdoor concerts as I could and sometimes danced to music in my living room.

I also practiced toning exercises—self-generated vocal sounds that have been found to manage pain and to reduce stress, insomnia, and symptoms of migraine. Sound therapy is based on the belief the body contains its own interlocking systems of vibrations, and that sound waves may be harnessed to balance the body's energy fields. Techniques vary, though the one I used is closest to that described in *The Mozart Effect*. Here, musician and educator Don Campbell directs the reader to find a comfortable position and to close his eyes. By using toning sounds such as "ah" and "ou," the reader is then told to visualize the discomfort released through one's own voice.

In time, I found I most enjoyed practicing toning while soaking in a warm bubble bath and varied the exercise by creating my own songs. Hearing the echoes bounce from the mirrored walls in the tiny room was mesmerizing. I devoted several evenings a month to this creative form of therapy. I always found the experience replenishing.

Books on tape were especially useful, too, since my concentration was scattered when I tried to read. Dr. Bernie Siegel's cancer tapes, especially those with music, are especially effective, as is John Kagat Zinn's series of *Stress Reduction* tapes, which are designed to induce a state of deep relaxation in which healing can occur.

There is a wide selection of inspirational tapes to choose from on the market. In addition to your local bookstore and library, check the hospitals, too; they often have collections of tapes to lend.

30

Acupuncture

Before each course of seventy-two-hour inpatient chemo-therapy, I received a one-hour acupuncture treatment at a nearby clinic. I then went from the acupuncturist to the hospital to begin chemotherapy treatment. I did this to prepare my system for the heavy doses of drugs I would be receiving.

Acupuncture, an ancient form of Chinese medicine that has been used for more than 4,500 years, is based on the idea that our energy or life force (known as "qi," pronounced chee) ebbs and flows with changes in our physical well-being. A balanced, free-flowing qi is said to generate good health, while energy channels that are blocked are believed to cause bodily malfunction and illness.

Practitioners strive to promote proper qi circulation by selectively placing tiny sterilized needles into the skin over specific body meridians (energy channels) to locate and release any such blockages. The needles may penetrate as little as a fraction of an inch, or as much as three to four inches, where a thick layer of fat or muscle exists. Aside from restoring balance to the body's energy channels, acupuncture is sometimes used as an effective anesthesia during surgery and to stimulate healing from many common ailments.

Acupuncture has gained steady prestige and official recognition in our country for its positive effects, and today over twelve thousand licensed acupuncturists and three thousand M.D.s perform it. A panel of experts at the National Institutes of Health concluded in a November 1997 report there was "clear evidence" that acupuncture eased chemotherapy-induced nausea and vomiting. Compared to conventional therapies, the panel found the side effects of acupuncture were few. Further evidence suggests acupuncture causes the release of natural pain-relieving endorphins.

It is difficult for me to evaluate the extent to which acupuncture ameliorated the extreme physical discomfort I experienced from four rounds of adriamycin, cisplatnum, and cytoxin intravenous injections. Because each of my chemotherapy treatments was preceded by acupuncture, I have no way of knowing how I would have done without it. Nonetheless, I found each acupuncture treatment to be painless and relaxing. And while the side effects of the chemotherapy were always rough, I kept reminding myself that it could be much worse. The integration of complementary therapies allowed me to feel confidence in the way I was addressing my illness.

All acupuncture consultations begin with an assessment of the patient's particular imbalance within the framework of Chinese medicine, but when there is cancer involvement, there are important differences. Typically the acupuncturist will pose a series of questions regarding the patient's responses to hot and cold and to taste. The tongue and the pulse points will be checked as well. All of this allows the practitioner to locate the energy blockages in the system and to identify which meridian points need stimulation to correct the imbalance.

When the illness a practitioner is treating is cancer, he or she needs to know if you are seeking treatment for pain or for chemotherapy-related distress. The practitioner also will want to know the kind of chemotherapy being used and the area it is meant to target. Like street maps broken down by neighborhoods, there are certain meridian or "acupoints" for each area of the body; knowing the correct ones to manipulate ensures that the procedure works with, not against, the bodily process.

Following the NIH's endorsement, the numbers of health insurers providing coverage for acupuncture has grown as the field, along with other natural therapies, has gained wider acceptance among health care professionals. Check with your insurance carrier regarding coverage. Your policy may require a doctor to authorize that it is medically necessary and may require a physician, rather than a licensed acupuncturist, to perform the procedure.

31

Seeking Joy

After being told by several physicians my remaining time was less than a year, I experienced an unexpected freedom. My life was being taken away from me but, oddly, handed back to me as well. I didn't have to worry any more about money or the future; about taking or not taking estrogen; or whether I had remembered to apply sunblock. It didn't matter if I cleaned out my cellar, spent too much money on a dress, or overindulged on oatmeal raisin cookies. I stopped fussing and micro-managing. I was going to die. But what was left of my life, for the first time ever, was entirely my own.

Believing I had few days ahead had the effect of making each one more spacious. My priorities shifted along with my view of the world. I deliberately sought all the joy I could muster. This was a time to take it all in, passionately—and I did.

I spent afternoons with my favorite people, took long car rides in the country, and picnicked in open fields. I visited art museums, read poetry while sipping Chardonnay in our canoe, sunbathed on sand dunes, soaked in long bubble baths, devoured boxes of fine chocolate, lighted candles, took walks in the park, and always made sure I had my friends around me.

I bought purple sweaters, a wetsuit for those cold swimming days, and browsed leisurely through upscale boutiques. I sang along at outdoor concerts, treated those I love to expensive dinners, and dunked in every nearby lake. When friends stopped by, we would often end up at the local ice cream stand sitting on the lawn licking peach frozen yogurt from a cone. I sampled all "36 flavors" of living, maxing out on joy to the fullest—then went back for more.

"Just as negative emotions produce negative chemical changes in the body," Norman Cousins instructed us a quarter century ago in *Anatomy of an Illness*, "so are positive emotions connected to positive changes. Joy triggers healthy endocrine functioning (including our immune system) and provides salubrious effects in our nervous and circulatory systems."

I discovered how full life becomes when death feels imminent. I learned how much there is to appreciate in the ordinary events of everyday life, and that joy comes from grabbing everything life offers. By actively seeking joy as I prepared for death, I entered into a new and more vibrant relationship with life.

If I Had My Life to Live Over, I Would Pick More Daisies

I'd like to make more mistakes next time
I'd relax. I would limber up.
I would be sillier than I've been this trip.
I would take fewer things seriously
I would take more chances
I would climb more mountains and swim more rivers
I would eat more ice cream and less beans
I would perhaps have more actual troubles,
but I'd have fewer imaginary ones.
You see, I'm one of those people who live sensibly
and sanely, hour after hour, day after day
Oh, I've had my moments, and if I had to do it again
I'd have more of them. In fact, I'd try to have nothing else.
Just moments one after the other, instead of
living so many years ahead of each day.
I've been one of those persons who never goes
anywhere without a thermometer, a hot water bottle,
a raincoat, and a parachute.

If I had to do it again, I would travel lighter than I have.
If I had my life to live over, I would start
barefoot earlier in the spring
and stay that way later in the fall.
I would go to more dances. I would ride
more merry-go-rounds
I would pick more daisies.

—NADINE STAIR

One of man's last freedoms is to choose one's
attitude in a given situation.
—DR. VIKTOR FRANKL,
MAN'S SEARCH FOR MEANING

Illuminated spiritual teachers die of heart disease and
cancer while cantankerous pessimists who smoke cigarettes
and eat lots of hamburgers sometimes live to be a hundred.
And all of us no matter how many bean sprouts we eat,
miles we run, affirmations we say, hours we meditate and
hard we pray, we are all going to die sometime. The question is not whether we will die, but how well we live.
—JOAN BORYSENKO, PH.D.

32

Forgiveness

My former training as a teacher and social worker stimulates my professional interest in keeping current with new self-help literature. A few months into my recovery I was able to concentrate once again and read. I soon became fascinated by all the attention then being given to the topic of forgiveness. It appeared everywhere, in almost everything I read.

Learning that the act of forgiveness can release cell toxicity and promote healing made a powerful impression.

It became increasingly evident to me how our bodies respond physically to the experience of anger and resentment: they close down. Our muscles tense; our chests feel tight and heavy; our breathing labors as stress and negativity act on our bodies.

Most interestingly, I discovered that our nervous systems are unable to distinguish between past and present events, so that whenever we mentally replay painful encounters and episodes, we feel the emotional impact of long-ago slights, injustices, and grievances as though they were happening *now*. Anger, in other words, knows no statute of limitations. Remembered resentment and hurt keep recycling themselves.

Understanding that the body reacts to every state of mind we experience, I realized that *holding on to anger was holding back my healing*. Having worked so hard to get better, I knew I didn't want the old anger inside me anymore. Like toxic waste, I needed to get rid of it. So I began to hone in on my life experience, to look openly at some past relationships and at lingering negative feelings I had never let go. Doing so motivated me to find a way to remove the anger I felt so that I would heal. I developed a method that I use to this day.

My Personal Forgiveness Program

1. I begin my forgiveness work after my morning meditation. This is a quiet period when I am

feeling centered. This precious time allows me to address forgiveness issues with a sense of peace rather than agitation.

2. Sitting in stillness, I visualize in my mind's eye the person I have harbored anger toward. I force myself to sit with the hurt and to feel it. Next I become aware of where in my body the anger shouts the loudest. I try not to dwell on specific scenes or conversations, for it is counterproductive to the forgiveness process. Doing so would pull me back into the death dance of fault and blame.

3. Next, I surrender the stored anger. I envision the anger as a cloud of black smoke. I observe the cloud being released from my heart center (or "chakra") and through the diaphragm as it is expelled with each rejuvenating breath I take.

4. I replace the black cloud with a visualized mass of healing white vapor. And then like a piece of driftwood being carried out to sea, the vapor drops past the horizon. It is gone.

5. I hold a feeling of peace in my heart as I simultaneously envision the person's face and move the healing white vapor around his or her being. I offer a blessing of goodwill to that person.

6. I repeat this technique several times a week.

The forgiveness process was a challenge at first. I struggled with it because stirring up feelings of resentment when we are in a weakened state is emotionally difficult

and may deplete needed energy stores. A part of me re-
sisted strongly and was crying out at every turn, "No way!"
But I also recalled reading somewhere that staying angry is
a way of letting another person live "rent-free" in your
head. And so I discovered that by practicing forgiveness, I
was enabling my own healing.

Months later, when I thought of the people in my life to
whom I had directed this technique I found that my feelings
toward them had changed. The anger and antagonism were
gone. A change had occurred. I felt freer, more energized,
less burdened. I no longer dwelled on negative feeling.

Repeating this process helped heal old wounds and
cleansed me. It was another way of keeping the positive
energy going. That is because forgiving is a conscious
choice. By activating my own will I was awakening my
capacity for inner peace and love and seeing beyond the
limits of another's personality—and my own. By practicing
forgiveness I was dismantling walls erected out of fear or
blame, freeing myself to see that other person, and myself,
anew. Forgiveness allowed me to reconfirm my feeling that
deep below our own egos, we are all the same.

It is said that charcoal does not become a diamond
unless it is exposed to pressure. In seeking your own for-
mula for forgiving, you can try thinking of a hot air balloon
tied down at four corners. Imagine you are forgiving each
person in your life who has hurt you as you unfasten each
side to release the cord holding it down. See yourself lifting
higher and higher as you rise above your anger.

Another method I use is the writing of a letter to the
person I hold anger toward. Sometimes I mail it or I crum-

ple it into a ball when I'm finished and burn it in the fireplace. I watch the process of the written words slowly disappearing into tiny embers. As the paper diminishes, I see my anger dissipate. My husband has his own method. He goes to the seashore with the name of the person he wants to forgive written on a folded piece of paper tucked into a bottle he then sends out to sea. By letting go of negative feelings we shift our thinking process and become more at peace with ourselves and the world.

My long recovery gave me a lot of time to think about my life and my own mistakes. It became important to me to close the circle of healing by looking inside to forgive myself for things I wish I had not said or done. Granting forgiveness to ourselves for past blunders is a cleansing process that allows for mind, body, and soul to become aligned. And it opens the body to fuller healing. Speaking out loud in front of a mirror, looking into your own eyes as you talk to yourself, or lighting a candle while reflecting on your past behavior can enhance the release of guilt, shame, and regret. Forgiving oneself and others is a sure path to emotional peace.

An Opportunity to Confront

A particular acquaintance, for whom I'd harbored bad feelings, was an old college classmate who lived thousands of miles away. She had been in those days a rude and insensitive person who had offended many, yet no one had had the courage to confront her. After all those years, the reverberation of her hurtful behavior still entered my consciousness whenever I thought of her.

Sometime after my cancer surgery, I got word of a college reunion. The rumor was Shelley was coming. Knowing this might be the only time I'd see her again, I wanted the opportunity to release my pent-up anger. This was my chance! Aside from wanting to connect with old friends, I felt an urgency to make the long drive to attend the reunion weekend. I knew this was the time to clean up old business.

The trip involved elaborate arrangements as I was recovering from chemo and felt very weak. I worried whether I'd be able to approach my classmate when I finally came face to face with her. I stayed awake nights feeling anxious about the encounter. But my motivation was strong. I had to go.

After an hour into the gathering, I saw Shelley saunter my way. As oldies music blared in the background, my palms began to sweat and my heart jumped. I quickly swallowed the contents of my wineglass and conjured up the courage to confront her. Wearing the same self-possessed grin I remembered, she positioned herself next to me, leaning her shoulder against the nearby wall. We awkwardly greeted one another and began to chat about the mundane things one talks about after a lapse of thirty years—where we were living, what our professional lives were, our husbands.

Then at what seemed to be the right moment, I placed my hand on her forearm and looked directly into her eyes. I was nonconfrontational but direct, and spoke from my heart. Shelley remained guarded, yet listened intently as I shared my lingering pain. When I finished she stood silently for a while, sipping gin and tonic. Then, following an uncomfortable silence, with her face angled toward the floor, she said, "I'm sorry. I've thought about my behavior in college and have suffered guilt. I was cruel in those days and don't know why."

She spoke openly for a while, sharing a grave family tragedy. Her only daughter had been born with a serious disability. She told me how her life had dramatically changed. Suddenly, Shelley became human to me, a person who suffered, too.

As she spoke, I felt as if a dark veil was lifting. I could feel my anger dissolving.

Overcome with a rush of compassion, we hugged for a moment. Then Shelley turned away to leave. As I watched her blend back into the smoky crowd I knew the negative feelings had disappeared for good. The pain was over.

The next morning Shelley appeared unexpectedly at my hotel door to say good-bye. We drank coffee together and recalled old times. As she left she invited me to visit her in Texas. I never saw her after that day, and probably never will again. But since that day I have been able to confront people who do or say things that are hurtful in a way I never could before. And I understand that in holding on to anger I cause myself needless pain.

....

What is not love is fear. Anger is one of fear's most potent forces. And it does exactly what fear wants it to do. It keeps us from receiving love at exactly the moment when we need it most.

—MARIANNE WILLIAMSON

Forgiveness is the act of admitting we
are exactly like other people.
—CHRISTINA BALDWIN,
LIFE'S COMPANION

There are two ways of spreading light: to be the
candle or the mirror that reflects it.
—EDITH WHARTON

33

Downtime

Even though you are handling things well and doing everything you can for your own well-being, you are still dealing with loss, pain, and sadness. Downtime is a designated time-out—a time set aside to allow yourself to feel and release those built-up emotions we all experience when going through a tumultuous period.

I experienced my share of rage and tears. Many a night, with my body sprawled across my bed and my face buried in a pillow, I'd scream at the top of my lungs.

Spending weeks confined in hospitals with multiple

roommates and their flustered families hovering near my bedside; having to smile to the families when they poked their heads through the curtains to say hello; adjusting my pain medication and getting comfortable only to have a new roommate wheeled into the room crying in pain from the discomfort; to say nothing of the strain of trying to steady my own frightened family and friends—all these took an enormous toll.

Hospitalization allows no space for downtime. I remember desperately wanting to be alone just to cry. During those vulnerable moments I resorted to journal writing, for it always felt too awkward to just let it all hang out with only a thin piece of cotton separating me from my sick neighbor. It would have been such a relief to have had a place to go to cry in private. Wouldn't it be grand to have insulated venting chambers in hospitals, so that patients could have a designated room to go to shed their tears in solitude?

Once you leave the hospital your depression may not fully dissipate. Taking time then to feel the sadness is vital—and different from just dwelling on your pain. Feeling sad doesn't mean feeling sorry for yourself. It means acknowledging what is happening. The reality of what you are facing needs to be honored.

I allowed myself ten minutes a day to feel down or to cry, always regaining my equilibrium when I was done. Allowing yourself to stay there does not promote healing; never allowing yourself to go there doesn't help either.

It is important to notify your family when you need time alone. When you want a time-out, close the door. I made a sign, "Taking Downtime," and hung it on the doorknob with a string of colored yarn when I didn't even want to speak.

Give yourself permission to be vulnerable. Taking time for a good cry or for pillow screaming can provide enormous release and is part of the healing process, too.

....

Tears are a river that take you somewhere . . . Tears lift your boat off the rocks, off dry ground, carrying it downriver to someplace new, someplace better.
—CLARISSA PINKOLA ESTES,
WOMEN WHO RUN WITH THE WOLVES

Be patient with all
that is unresolved
And try to love
the questions themselves
Do not seek
for the answers that
cannot be given
For you would not
be able to live them
And the point is to
live everything
Live the questions
now
And Perhaps
without

knowing it
You will
live along
someday
into the answers.
—RAINER MARIA RILKE,
LETTERS TO A YOUNG POET

34

Compassion

I have always cherished the friends I have had throughout my lifetime. During my struggle I was fortunate indeed
to be supported by so many compassionate souls.

After my diagnosis, however, there were some surprises.
Some of my strongest supporters turned out to be people
whom I never would have predicted would be there, while
others who professed to be tried and true could not handle
the trauma and walked away. A few were brave enough to
express their fears to me honestly, while others remained

silent and quietly disappeared. Each abandonment was profoundly painful and it was hard not to take it personally. I fought not to allow the loss to set me back.

I eventually came to understand that when friends deal with cancer, they confront the most private, primal, and frightened parts of themselves. Cancer makes us afraid. It challenges us to live up to *the way we'd like to think we'd behave in crisis.* We are made to confront losses all over again. We have to face up to the stark reality of our own mortality.

Our friends worry they'll disappoint us, and themselves. That they'll reveal their inadequacies. They worry: Am I going to be brought down by this emotionally? Am I going to be called upon too often? Will it be too upsetting for me? Will I be able to fulfill the role of a good friend? Am I doing this right? Will I know what to say? Will I make her feel worse? And . . . will I be next?

I reached a milestone in my emotional growth when I was finally able to let go of the hurt. With time I learned compassion. Compassion for the friends who could not face their own mortality and turned away. Compassion for the friends who could not trust themselves. Compassion for the doctors who could not look me in the eye. And compassion for the nurses who thought they knew what was best for me by keeping the frightening facts from me—the medical literature I needed to begin to fight for my life.

With time I was able to reach a place inside myself where anger and judgment were pushed aside, where pain was released and replaced by empathy for another soul. When I think about the friends who abandoned me, my feelings are complex. For what my experience has taught has truly enlarged my being, while fear has shrunk theirs. I hope they, too, will find their peace.

The following story from the Reverend Mary Manin Morrissey, author of *Building Your Field of Dreams*, helped guide me.

A rabbi was giving instruction to some children, when he posed this question: "How do you know the night is over and the day has come?" Puzzled, the children took some time to answer. Then one of them ventured, "You know the night is over and the day has come when, at dawn, you look out at a tree, and you can tell whether it is an apple or a pear tree." The rabbi acknowledged this response, but repeated the question. A second student offered, "You know the night is over and the day has come when you see an animal in the distance, and you can tell whether it is a donkey or a horse." The rabbi acknowledged this response too, then repeated the question. At this the students, too puzzled to know how to answer, asked the rabbi to solve the dilemma he had posed. The rabbi said, "You know the night is over and the day has come when you look into the eyes of any human being, and you see there your brother or your sister; for, if you do not see your brother or your sister, it is still night—the day hasn't come."

Friendship with oneself is all important; without it we
cannot be friends with anyone else in the world.
—FLORENCE NIGHTINGALE

It is an illusion that we are in separate bodies.
—ALBERT EINSTEIN

Spiritual energy brings compassion into the real world.
With compassion, we see benevolently our own human
condition and the condition of our fellow beings. We drop
prejudice. We withhold judgment.
—CHRISTINA BALDWIN,
LIFE'S COMPANION

35

Create a Sanctuary

During my time of healing I found I needed to bring more beauty into my life, to surround myself with attractive objects, cozy fabrics, beloved memorabilia, and talismans from nature that would connect me to the outdoors. Like a nature sanctuary, where birds and wildlife take refuge in safety from hunters, I was moved to create a personal space that would put me beyond the long reach of illness.

Illness is a time when you need more quiet, more serenity, and a healthy escape from the chaos of the outside world. The world around us fills our heads constantly with its technological messages; the airwaves and print media can bombard us with negative data that can overwhelm. My sanctuary evolved out of my need to block out the constant media drone, to insulate myself from the world and encourage a calm state of being.

I brought nature inside my house—delicate seashells, sea glass washed ashore, and autumn hydrangeas whose rich color had been deepened by the sudden cold. I found pine needles and eucalyptus leaves. Breathing in their healthy scents, I envisioned my lungs opening and cleaning my cells.

I framed favorite poems and meaningful pictures—my childhood birthday parties, high school picnics at the beach, and my wedding. I brought in whatever I thought would raise my spirits and open me to more healing in my life. I changed the lighting to a softer hue and lit tea candles in colored jars. I filled silver bowls with lavender potpourri and covered oversized pillows with luxurious fabrics. I chose blue so that my spirit could wander, red so it could blaze with hope, and green so my soul could rest. My sanctuary made me feel warm and secure. It was a sacred place that sustained me.

In Japan each home contains an altar, a special corner of beauty. Similarly, your sanctuary need be no larger than a space in your bedroom or a tabletop covered by a pretty cloth. Try to find a private niche in a home office, den, or enclosed porch that you can transform into your own holy ground. There are many gates to the sacred and they can be as diverse as we need them to be.

Make your space a personal temple. Bring to it your favorite books, tapes, and a CD player. Sports trophies, family albums, a painting, or armed service decorations, photographs of places you wish to visit when this is all behind you, boxes of assorted chocolates, and handmade crafts—anything that has special meaning for you and makes your heart sing. Create a retreat that lifts you like music—and will draw you back again and again.

....

Never lose an opportunity to see anything beautiful.
Beauty is God's handwriting.
—CHARLES KINGSLEY, *CRISP TOASTS*, WILLIAM R.
EVANS III AND ANDREW FROTHINGHAM, EDITORS

Just as the silent snow settles in
covering rough edges and filling empty spaces
So may peace settle upon our lives
And wrap us in beauty.
—UNKNOWN

Beauty is an ecstasy. It is as simple as hunger.
—SOMERSET MAUGHAM, *CAKES AND ALE*

....

36

Therapeutic Massage

Just as therapeutic touch is proving to be a modality that can ease discomfort and promote well-being, documented research shows that massage therapy can alter neuropeptides, thereby increasing neural activity and functioning and releasing body toxins. Massage is also said to stimulate the brain's creation of natural, pain-relieving endorphins, which perhaps explains why we generally feel better and more tranquil following a massage.

I consulted first with my physicians to make sure massage was not contraindicated, and then interviewed certified massage therapists over the telephone. I asked the practitioners about their experience working with cancer patients, about the kind of therapeutic massage techniques they used, and how the therapy would be tailored to accommodate my particular circumstances.

This is *very* important. Some practitioners feel that rubbing muscle tissue in an area where there are a lot of cancer cells can release carcinogens into the bloodstream. I also knew that more vigorous approaches would be wrong for me, as I could tolerate only light pressure. I selected a licensed female practitioner who was willing to come to my home. In addition I called my insurance company regarding coverage. Some companies consider massage therapy to be an adjunct form of medical treatment.

The routine that the therapist and I evolved extends to this day. She brings an electric blanket and a heating pad to warm the towels that will be used. She fills the room with classical music, in the winter turns up the thermostat in the house to eighty degrees, dims the light, and asks me to chose an aromatic oil.

I always ask the therapist to gently massage the area *around* my surgical scar to help regenerate the nerves and help relieve the numbness in the tissue that I still feel. It took many months following my surgeries and the long stretch of postoperative therapies for my bruised and abused body to feel anything like normal. I had been cut and radiated, chest tubes had hung out of my side, broken ribs had caused great discomfort, and I now lived with a hundred metal clips placed permanently around my heart to keep my rebuilt chest wall intact. My body was both numb and hypersensitive. The discomfort was continuous. With time it became more tolerable. After my doctor gave the go-ahead, I found the massage therapy I received helped stretch tissue and increase my range of motion, enhancing the overall healing.

As the massage therapist delicately manipulates the muscles and applies almost imperceptible pressure to the soft tissue areas, time feels suspended. I listen to the gentle flow of my breathing. I appreciate the stillness of the room. I focus on my body's response, as the massage therapist coaxes the nerves and tissue to revive. And when the hour is finished, I always remember to drink a lot of spring water to help release the body toxins.

I find massage to be both relaxing and therapeutic, an effect that usually lasts several days. I still indulge in a massage once a month, a luxury and a continuing source of well-being.

37

Humor

I have a favorite cartoon created by the illustrator Ed Stein. A man is lying in a hospital bed, his head wrapped in bandages, connected to an IV, covers pulled to his chin, a weary, feverish look on his face. The entire wall of his room is papered with a checkerboard of X rays—of his skull, spine, hands, feet, chest, and hip bone—it's all there. Beside him stands a chipper-looking physician, who asks: "Let's try this another way. What *doesn't* hurt?"

Today that cartoon brings a smile to my face but not so long ago, when every part of me was in pain, laughter did not come as easily. Even so, knowing that emotions affect chemical production in the body and that continual feelings of despair and self-pity can be toxic, I was motivated to make space for *lighter times*.

As individuals we tend to experience humor cognitively, emotionally, and physically. So many of life's mundane experiences can be viewed as humorous. By keeping myself open I was often amused, even in my darkest times.

One afternoon not long after we put our house up for sale, Channah, my energy healer, arrived for her usual session. We decided to take advantage of the good weather and move outdoors to the back porch. As I lay on a lounge chair, she danced around me reciting biblical passages, with music blaring, then kneeled down over me to administer healing touch to my forehead. At just that moment I heard someone say "Oh, *excuse* us! We didn't know anybody was here." I sat up to look into the astonished face of the Realtor, who had arrived unannounced with two eager clients to see our house and was now backing away. I'm sure they didn't know what to think; I was lying prone and Channah was practically on top of me. I was deeply flustered, but then burst into loud laughter.

Many of the life-enhancing effects of laughter are well documented. Laughter reduces serum cortisol, a hormone released during the stress response and increases immunoglobin A, an antibody that helps fight upper respiratory disease. Laughter increases our pain threshold, our energy level, our heart and pulse rates, and stimulates the internal organs: consider the physiological effect on our bodies that comes from a good belly laugh. Isn't it remarkable to think that a smile or a mere chuckle can cause changes in our biochemical state?

Although the full effect of humor on the immune system is not fully understood, we do know from studies that humor helps us by replacing distressing emotions with pleasurable ones. As Dr. Steve Sultanoff, who studies the role therapeutic humor plays in healing, explains, "Humor and distressing emotions cannot occupy the same psychological space. You cannot feel angry, depressed, anxious, guilty, or resentful and experience humor at the same time." Think how many of us have experienced situations when we've been angry and suddenly someone says or does something funny, he continues. "A typical response is, 'Don't make me laugh. I want to be angry.' Intuitively we know that we cannot maintain distress and experience humor simultaneously."

There will be more news on the healing power of humor to come. The UCLA School of Medicine has just received a research grant from the Comedy Central Network to learn how to best use humor to treat pain and disease. Humor will be studied as a tool to instruct and educate patients on health issues and as a form of therapy to ease the emotional problems that can result from illness. Fittingly, the five-year project is called "RX Laughter."

The first time I laughed after I learned I had cancer was during a neighbor's barbecue. There was such ease and merriment as we chatted with the other guests in their beautiful backyard, I laughed out loud. It felt good. Until then I had thought I had forgotten how to laugh. Later on, I would chuckle at some of the funny cards I received. To add a note of humor to my hospital room, I hung a turquoise T-shirt a girlfriend had given me on the wall that read, "Still crazy after all these years." While I was recovering at home, my husband served me as a waiter with a towel over his forearm speaking in broken French. And for a diversion I rented funny movies and upbeat videos. Laughter altered my mood and helped me escape temporarily. Laughter is certainly one of the best medicines.

A good laugh is as good as prayer sometimes.
—L. M. MONTGOMERY,
RILLA OF INGLESIDE

A merry heart doeth good like a medicine.
—DR. LEE BERK, LOMA LINDA UNIVERSITY
SCHOOLS OF MEDICINE AND PUBLIC HEALTH,
WWW.HUMORPROJECT.COM

He who laughs, lasts!
—MARY PETTIBONE POOLE,
A GLASS EYE AT A KEYHOLE

38

Hypnosis

Hypnosis can be a valuable tool for reducing anxiety and minor pain, ending panic, overcoming phobias, and insulating oneself against stress. Contrary to what many believe, an unwilling subject cannot be hypnotized, nor is it something that a practitioner "does" to a subject. Those who remember the *Manchurian Candidate* may be surprised to know that hypnosis was not born with the Cold War. Rather, hypnosis is several thousand years old. In ancient times, so-called sleep temples were places where troubled

Greeks and Romans could seek help with their physical and emotional ailments.

Hypnosis is an altered state of consciousness, a way of relaxing into a deepened state of concentration. What you hear from your hypnotist, together with positive images you call to mind, replace the negative images stored in your subconscious with associations that are more comforting and reassuring. If administered by a medically trained hypnotist, this therapy can be most effective.

I was very anxious about beginning cancer treatment. I knew I was in for a long haul and recognized I had to deal with my underlying fears. A few weeks before my scheduled surgery, I asked my doctor for a referral. He sent me to a psychologist specializing in hypnotherapy at the Mind Body Clinic at Deaconess Hospital in Boston. I was told the hypnotherapist could guide me through the steps of hypnosis or teach me how to perform the techniques myself.

During my initial session I shared my fears. I talked about my fear of surgery and pain, my anxiety concerning hair loss and incapacitation. I spoke about what my illness was going to do to my family. I talked about my fear of death.

I left the practitioner's office with a tape describing how I could experience a hypnotic state. The tape described breathing, focusing, and relaxation techniques. At home when I played the tape I closed my eyes and focused on alleviating my fears. The session and tape were both helpful and I am glad I included the visit in my presurgery plan, although I did not go further with it. By this time I felt I had done all I could. I had prepared myself and felt it was time to put into practice everything I had learned about visualization, guided imagery, and meditation. I used my experience with hypnosis to enhance my visualization and meditation work.

Hypnosis has been shown to be an effective tool and worth trying for treating the anxiety attached to hospitalization or to counteract the fear that can intensify pain and complicate healing. If you decide to look into this modality, check credentials carefully. My preference is someone who has a medical background. In some instances, health insurers will provide benefits for sessions performed by licensed professionals.

39

Vital References

The following resources are those I personally used. I highly recommend their services.

The American Cancer Society is a national organization that offers tremendous assistance. It can be reached by calling 800-Cancer, or (800) 227-2345, the Information Service number of the National Institutes of Cancer. Valuable information on all aspects of cancer is provided free of charge. The comprehensive literature ranges from how to deal with nutrition and dietary intake to dealing with social issues and family concerns. I read the booklets from cover to cover.

Cancer Care is a national nonprofit organization based

in New York City. It offers support for cancer patients and their families. There are national teleconferencing services, seminars, booklets, and phone support groups, all free of charge. Social workers are available by phone to answer questions. Financial planning seminars at no cost are offered for residents of New York, New Jersey, and Connecticut. The number is (800) 813-HOPE. In Manhattan, call (212) 302-2400, or use the website (*www.cancercare.org*).

The Wellness Community is a psycho-social and educational organization that offers support to cancer patients, friends, and families. Gilda Radner, the well-known comedienne who struggled and lost her battle with ovarian cancer, wrote appreciatively about her experiences there in her memoir, *It's Always Something.*

There are twenty Wellness Communities in the United States and each one has ongoing support groups with workshops ranging from nutrition to yoga. Their services are offered at no charge. I attended many of their programs and admire the outstanding work they do. The national headquarters, which may be reached at (888) 793-9355, can inform you as to whether there is an organization in your area.

The Internet. In addition to using the Internet to access current health information covering many cancer types and the newest protocols available, I participate in various chat rooms, another excellent way to network or find group support.

I do this simply by typing in "cancer" on the top bar of my screen. When the boxed directory list appears on the screen, I click on to "chat rooms," where I can read and post messages on "bulletin boards." In responding to some-one else's message, I have the option of replying to the person privately by e-mail or of leaving a message on the chat board the person may open whenever she or he goes back into the message board area. A wonderful feature of chat rooms is that you can also *ask* questions by posting a topic on a subject of your choice.

The computer is a valuable resource putting useful data at one's fingertips. I try to keep current with the ongoing research on nutrition, health care, and cancer studies.

Financial Supports are available to help meet the needs of paying for the various components of cancer treatment. The organizations listed above, along with others like the United Way ([800] 411-UWAY), and government programs like Medicare and the Hill-Burton Compensated Services Program, can help qualified individuals find services at little or no cost.

While health insurance covers most treatment costs, including the hospital and physicians' bills, you may need to take time off from your work for some period while you recover and undergo postsurgical treatment. Disability benefits, whether from private insurers or from public entitlements, vary markedly. Meeting out-of-pocket expenses not usually covered by insurance (medication, transportation, home care, and child care) as well as ordinary monthly expenses—the mortgage, fuel, food, and electricity—can become difficult under these circumstances. To find relief:

- Review your insurance policy to understand your coverage.

- Speak to the Personnel or Human Resources director at your place of employment and to a hospital or community social worker to determine what you are entitled to collect.
- Phone your local cancer society chapter to learn about community supports.
- Check the Yellow Pages of your phone directory for listings of nearby social service organizations and for listings of state and local government agencies. Their representatives can describe the various entitlements and services you may be eligible to receive, including the enrollment procedures required.

The Internet is another tool that can help you investigate these services. Cancer Care's "Money Matters" section, located in its Helping Hand Resource Database, lists by state and by region various services that can help you with financial entitlements and benefits, direct financial assistance, assistance for medications, and health insurance information.

Similarly, government agency home pages (i.e., the Social Security Administration Medicare Benefits Program, the U.S. Department of Health and Human Services, and Medicaid Consumer Information for state-administered health insurance programs) may also be consulted.

Other invaluable services are listed on Resource pages at the end of this book. Taking advantage of the wealth of resources that exist out there can offer enormous support and comfort during the trying journey.

40

Taking Care

of Business

I realized that practicing the *art of positive thinking* did not negate the practical need to get my affairs in order. I found a lawyer who helped me prepare a will. I created a list, dividing my jewelry and other possessions among family and loved ones. I wrote letters to old high-school buddies and contacted dear friends. I took care of appropriate concerns.

My attorney also helped me prepare three key documents: a durable power of attorney, a health care proxy, and a living will. The names of these documents may vary from state to state.

By preparing a power of attorney I was designating someone I trusted to act on my behalf in financial matters. A *durable* power of attorney becomes effective immediately upon signature and *stays* in effect if and when the principal becomes incapacitated, or is no longer able to make informed decisions. A general, or broad, power of attorney, on the other hand, becomes invalid when the principal becomes incapacitated. The durable power of attorney, then, is the instrument that anticipates the needs associated with serious illness.

A health care proxy allowed me to designate a person (or agent) to make medical decisions in the event I was not able to do so. It goes into effect only after a patient becomes incapacitated. Until such a time, I would continue to have the right to make my own decisions, as well as to change or limit the conditions of the proxy if I chose. The health care proxy I prepared was signed and dated before two witnesses. I then informed my doctors and left copies in my medical charts.

A living will described the health care I wanted were life-sustaining treatments in the event of imminent death to become necessary. It is *not* a substitute for the more flexible health care proxy because this written evidence of my wishes would supersede any end-of-life decisions my proxy (or agent) made on my behalf. Like the proxy, my living will was signed and witnessed. I gave a copy to my physician to keep in my file.

It is always worthwhile to make one's wishes known to loved ones before a crisis. Your health care proxy, along with other family members, can be under great emotional strain. It is easier to make any critical decisions that must be made when those doing so feel confidence that what they are doing is what you would have wanted. Because death sometimes is tragically unexpected, it is always a good idea, no matter what one's age or condition of health, for your family to have a conversation about heroic interventions and end-of-life preparations.

Standard legal documents are available from your state's Department of Health, in some banks or other financial institutions, and in legal stationery stores. You may also contact Choice in Dying by phone ([800] 989-WILL), in writing (Suite 10001, 200 Varick Street, New York, NY 10014) or on-line (*www.choices.org*). This advocacy organization provides information concerning patient's rights regarding medical treatments, living wills, and other legal options when death is near. They can explain how to prepare and execute living wills and health care proxy documents. Be sure to request the documents for your state.

The Institute for Certified Financial Planners, a trade association based in Denver, Colorado, can provide names of members who specialize in assisting people with serious illness. To help decide which planner might best meet your personal needs, call (800) 282-7526.

Taking control of business allowed me to take charge of a part of my life that I could control. Getting my affairs in place offered a certain comfort.

Hope is an orientation of spirit, an orientation of the heart. It is not the conviction that something will turn out well, but the certainty that something makes sense regardless of how it turns out.

—VACLAV HAVEL

41

Stay Positive, Persistent,

and Persevere

After I was diagnosed with cancer I did everything I could to ensure the best possible outcome. That began with making sure I selected a hospital and medical team I felt confident about, and I will always be profoundly grateful to the physicians, nurses, therapists, social workers, and medical technicians who treated me. But when their job was finished, *it was up to me to continue the work.*

Throughout my ordeal, I kept reminding myself that doctors merely practice medicine. I respected the mind/body connection and realized the ability to heal ourselves is boundless. Hippocrates, the father of medicine, understood this when he declared: "Patient heal thyself."

I tried to utilize every resource, every appropriate medical treatment, and every bit of mental discipline I had during my battle. I wanted to live. In the process of fighting for my life, I never gave up hope, never stopped taking chances, never stopped trying new things. If we don't take risks, I once read, we will never experience the joy that comes from learning *we can change ourselves* and our outcome.

I remember how my mother used to say when I was a child, in the words of Lincoln, "This too shall pass." I never realized the impact these words would one day have on my life. Some days I recited them from morning till night, just trying to make it through, searching for a crack of light in the cold thin darkness.

My mother's spirit remains with me, and so much more, for without the gift of her extraordinary tenacity I might well have given up. My other model was Norman Cousins, known for his self-cure from a debilitating illness through a program of laughter and vitamin C. During my healing I read and reread and even included on my personal tape this particular passage from his remarkable *Anatomy of an Illness:*

> I have learned never to underestimate the capacity of the human mind and body to regenerate even when the prospects seem most wretched. The life force may be the least understood force on earth. William James said that "human beings tend to live too far within

self imposed limits." It is possible that these limits will recede when we respect more fully the natural drive of the human mind and body toward perfectibility and regeneration. Protecting and cherishing that natural drive may well represent the finest exercise of human freedom.

As the lives of each of us dramatically unfold and we begin to discover our unique purpose here, we must honor the diverse healings that come to us in so many different forms.

While driven in our quest for physical health, let us never discount the magnitude of an emotional or spiritual healing. For just as a flower opens to the morning sun, we must stay attuned to the light, so we, too, can be receptive to the grand universal gifts.

No, I am not living the life I had planned, but with boundless gratitude I live the life that was waiting for me— and in the process, I hope to continue to inspire others so they, too, can learn to harness their skills to empower themselves and begin to heal.

As you continue to embrace the mystery of life's challenges, may you find the courage to persevere on your journey toward wellness, and may you be blessed with inner peace. I wish you serene moments, joyful experiences, and new beginnings.

I got well by talking. Death could not get a word in
edgewise, grew discouraged, and traveled on.
—LOUISE ERDRICH, *TRACKS*

I will not live in fear
of falling or catching fire
I choose to inhabit my days
to allow my living to open me
to make me less afraid, more accessible
to loosen my heart
Until it becomes a wing
A torch. A promise.
I choose to risk my insignificance;
to live so that which comes to me as seed
goes to the next as blossom
and that which comes to me as blossom
goes on to fruit.
—DAWNA MARKOVA,
I WILL NOT DIE AN UNLIVED LIFE

Notes

Page 41   *These people had the quality of* Caryle Hirshberg and Marc Ian Barasch, *Remarkable Recovery: What Extraordinary Healings Tell Us About Getting Well and Staying Well*, New York: Berkley Publishing Group, 1996, p. 27.

Page 42   *The swords of battle* Stephen Jay Gould, "The Median Isn't the Message," On-line at *www.cancerguide.org/ median_msg.html*.

Page 55   *an excitation of nerve cells* Michael Samuels, M.D., *Healing with the Mind's Eye: A Guide for Using Imagery and Visions for Personal Growth and Healing*, New York: Summit Books, 1990, p. 9.

Page 112   *According to one report* Michael Lloyd, "Writing Myself," *Gay Chicago Magazine*, August 19–29, 1999: 22.

Page 120   *surgical patients who could view trees* Anne Raver, "Gardens That Harness Nature's Healing Powers," *New York Times*, June 25, 2000, p. 6.

Page 128   *"Faith empowers science . . ."* Larry Dossey, M.D., *Healing Words: The Power of Prayer and the Practice of Medicine*, San Francisco: HarperCollins, 1993, p. 54.

Page 129   *"To be healed . . ."* Lewis Mehl-Madrona, M.D., *Coyote Medicine: Lessons from Native American Healing*, New York: Simon & Schuster, 1997, p. 129.

Page 131   *a field of palpable energy* George Leonard and Michael Murphy, *The Life We Are Given: A Daily Program for Realizing the Potential of Body, Mind, Heart, and Soul*, New York: Putnam Publishing Company, 1995, pp. 66–67.

Page 139   *Recent studies published* "Foods That Fight Disease: Green Tea," *Health* magazine, San Francisco: December 4, 1997, p. 8.

Page 141   *Legumes have a molecule* "Cancer and Health," *Rider College Bulletin*, Lawrenceville, N.J.: 1986, p. 4.

Page 142   *large intakes of broccoli* "Foods That Fight Disease: Broccoli and Cabbage, *Health* magazine, December 4, 1997, p. 9.

Page 150   *the three most nutritious fruits* Andrew Weil, M.D., "The Power of Produce," *Dr. Andrew Weil's Self Healing Newsletter*, Watertown, Mass.: July 1999, p. 1.

Page 163   At *Columbia Presbyterian Medical* Peggy Huddleston, *Prepare for Surgery, Heal Faster*, Cambridge, Mass.: Angel River Press, p. 128.

Page 163   *the journal* Cancer *concluded* "Complementary Care for Cancer," *Dr. Andrew Weil's Self Healing Newsletter*, January 1998, p. 6.

Page 165   *Throughout time man* "Sound Healing," *Dr. Andrew Weil's Self Healing Newsletter*, February 1998, p. 1.

Page 167   *By using toning sounds* Don Campbell, *The Mozart Effect: Tapping the Power of Music to Heal the Body, Strengthen the Mind, and Unlock the Spirit*, New York: Avon Books, 1997, p. 67.

Page 169   *A panel of experts* "NIH Panel Research Endorses Acupuncture," *Dr. Andrew Weil's Self Healing Newsletter*, January 1998, p. 7.

Page 173   *"Just as negative emotions . . ."* Norman Cousins, *Anatomy of an Illness: As Perceived by the Patient*, New York: W. W. Norton, 1979, p. 56.

Page 201   *As Dr. Steve Sultanoff* "Questions and Answers About Therapeutic Humor," On-line at *http://www.aath.org*.

Page 215   *I have learned never* Cousins, p. 85.

Bibliography

All my life I have collected quotations from a vast array of sources—literature, magazines, even greeting cards. Copied down on odd paper scraps or neatly clipped before pasting into my journals, returning to my quotations is like rummaging through an attic and happening upon treasures. Many of them are included in this book. In addition, I have been inspired by numerous anthologies. Among these are *The New Beacon Book of Quotations by Women* by Rosalie Maggio (Boston: Beacon Press, 1996) and *And I Quote: The Definitive Collection of Quotes, Sayings, and Jokes for the Contemporary Speechmaker* by Ashton Applewhite, William R. Evans III, and Andrew Frothingham (New York: St. Martin's Press, 1992).

"Acupuncture: New Uses for an Ancient Art." *Dr. Andrew Weil's Self Healing Newsletter*, April 1998: 2–3.

Alexander, Skye. "The Power of Prayer." *Earth Star*, April/May 1998: 25–26.

"The Anti-Cancer Diet." *Dr. Andrew Weil's Self Healing Newsletter*, January 1997: 1–3.

"The Art of Breathing." *Dr. Andrew Weil's Self Healing Newsletter*, May 1998: 1, 6–7.

Benson, Herbert, M.D. *Timeless Healing: The Power and Biology of Belief*. New York: Scribner, 1996.

Byrd, R. C. "Positive Therapeutic Effects of Intercessory Prayer in a Coronary Care Population." *Southern Medical Journal* 81, no. 7 (1988).

Campbell, Don. *The Mozart Effect: Tapping the Power of Music to Heal the Body, Strengthen the Mind, and Unlock the Spirit*. New York: Avon Books, 1997.

"Can Spirituality Heal?" *Dr. Andrew Weil's Self Healing Newsletter*, January 2000: 8.

Cancer Care Helping Hand Resource Database [On-line]. Available HTTP: *http://www.cancercare.orghhrd/hhrd_financial/htm*.

"Cancer and Health." *Rider College Bulletin* 2, no. 6 (1986): 4.

Casarjian, Robin. *Forgiveness: A Bold Choice for a Peaceful Heart*. New York: Bantam, 1992.

"Chemotherapy: Myth and Reality for Older Patients." *Focus on Healthy Aging*, Mt. Sinai School of Medicine 2, no. 10 (October 1999): 4–5.

"Complementary Care for Cancer." *Dr. Andrew Weil's Self Healing Newsletter*, January 1998: 1, 6–7.

Consumer Reports on Health. "How to Find a Good Surgeon." June 2000: 5.

Cousins, Norman. *Anatomy of an Illness: As Perceived by the Patient*. New York: W. W. Norton, 1979.

"Decisions Resource Report." *New Age Journal*, April, 1997.

Dion, Susan, Ph.D. *Write Now: Maintaining a Creative Spirit While Homebound and Ill*. Carneys Point, N.J.: Puffin Foundation Ltd., 1993.

Dold, Catherine. "Acupuncture: Getting the Point," *IONS: Noetic Science Review*, August–November 1999: 9.

Dossey, Larry, M.D. *Healing Words: The Power of Prayer and the Practice of Medicine*. San Francisco: HarperCollins, 1993.

"Energy Medicine: A New Frontier." *Dr. Andrew Weil's Self Healing Newsletter*, October 2000: 1, 6.

"Foods That Fight Disease: Broccoli and Cabbage." *Health* magazine, December 4, 1997: 9.

"Foods That Fight Disease: Green Tea," *Health* magazine, December 4, 1997: 8.

"Ginger and Chemo May Not Mix," *Environmental Nutrition* 19, no. 9 (September 1996): 2.

Gordon, Thomas. *Parent Effectiveness Training: The Tested New Way to Raise Responsible Children*. New York: Peter H. Wyden, 1970.

————. *Leadership Training: The No-Lose Way to Release the Productive Potential of People*. New York: Wyden Books, 1977.

Gould, Stephen Jay. "The Median Isn't the Message" [On-line]. Available HTTP: *www.cancerguide.org/median_msg.html*.

Hanh, Thich Nhat. *The Miracle of Mindfulness: A Manual on Meditation*. Boston: Beacon Press, 1987.

"Healing with the Creative Arts." *Dr. Andrew Weil's Self Healing Newsletter*, May 2000: 1, 6–7.

"The Healing Power of Green Tea." *Dr. Andrew Weil's Self Healing Newsletter*, October 1998: 2.

"Healing Touch." *Dr. Andrew Weil's Self Healing Newsletter*, October 2000: 7.

Hirshberg, Caryle, and Marc Barasch, *Remarkable Recovery: What Extraordinary Healings Tell Us About Getting Well and Staying Well*. New York: Berkley Publishing Group, 1996.

Huddleston, Peggy. *Prepare for Surgery, Heal Faster: A Guide to Mind-Body Techniques*. Cambridge, Mass.: Angel River Press, 1996.

Kabat-Zinn, Jon. *Full Catastrophe Living: Using the Wisdom of Your Body and Mind to Face Illness*. New York: Delacorte, 1990.

————. *Wherever You Go, There You Are: Mindfulness Meditation in Everyday Life*. New York: Hyperion, 1994.

Kesten, Deborah. *Feeding the Body, Nourishing the Soul: The Essentials of Eating for Physical, Emotional, and Spiritual Well-Being*. Berkeley, Calif.: Conari Press, 1997.

Klein, Allen. "Who Says Humor Heals?" [On-line]. Available HTTP: *http://members.aol.com/_ht_a/USmile2743/humor.humor_heals.html.*

Knight, Bryan, "Hypnotherapy," in Janet Gotkin and Kate Pages, eds., *HealthInform's Resource Guide to Alternative Health: An Annual Directory of Information Sources on Alternative and Complementary Therapies.* Montrose, N.Y.: HealthInform, 1997.

Koenig, Harold, M.D. *The Healing Power of Faith: Science Explores Medicine's Last Frontier.* New York: Simon & Schuster, 1999.

Krieger, Delores. *The Therapeutic Touch.* New York: Fireside Press, 1979.

Lee, Roberta, M.D. "Guided Imagery as Supportive Therapy in Cancer Treatment." *Alternative Medicine Alert* 2, no. 6 (June 1999): 61–64.

Leeds, Dorothy. *The Seven Powers of Questions: Secrets to Successful Communication in Life and Work.* New York: Berkley Publishing Group, 2000.

Leonard, George, and Michael Murphy. *The Life We Are Given: A Daily Program for Realizing the Potential of Body, Mind, Heart, and Soul.* New York: Jeremy Tarcher/Putnam Publishing Group, 1995.

Lerner, Michael. *Choices in Healing: Integrating the Best of Conventional and Complementary Approaches to Cancer.* Cambridge, Mass.: MIT Press, 1994.

LeShan, Lawrence. *Cancer as a Turning Point: A Handbook for People with Cancer, Their Families, and Health Professionals.* New York: Plume, 1994.

Levine, Stephen. *A Year to Live: How to Live Your Life as If It Were Your Last.* New York: Bell Tower/Harmony Books, 1997.

————. "To Live Before I Die." *New Age Journal*, March/April 1997, pp. 72–77.

Lloyd, Michael. "Writing Myself." *Gay Chicago Magazine*, no. 33, August 19–29, 1999: 21–22.

Madison, Deborah. *Vegetarian Cooking for Everyone.* New York: Broadway Books, 1997.

"Making the Most of Meditation." *Dr. Andrew Weil's Self Healing Newsletter*, June 2000: 2–3.

"Making a Place for Spirituality." *Harvard Health Letter* 23, no. 4 (February 1998): 1–3.

Mehl-Madrona, Lewis, M.D. *Coyote Medicine: Lessons from Native American Healing.* New York: Simon & Schuster, 1997.

Myss, Carolyn. *Anatomy of a Spirit: The Seven Stages of Power and Healing.* New York: Harmony Books, 1996.

"NIH Panel Research Endorses Acupuncture." *Dr. Andrew Weil's Self Healing Newsletter*, January 1998: 3.

"The Power of Produce." *Dr. Andrew Weil's Self Healing Newsletter*, July 1999: 1.

"'Prayer Is Good Medicine,' says Dr. Dossey." *Medicine and Prayer: The Newsletter of the Santa Fe Institute for Medicine and Prayer*, December, January 1997: 1–2.

"Protecting Against Colon Cancer." *Dr. Andrew Weil's Self Healing Newsletter*, January 2000: 6–7.

"Questions and Answers About Therapeutic Humor." American Association for Therapeutic Humor [On-line]. Available HTTP: *http://www.aath.org*.

Raver, Anne. "Gardens That Harness Nature's Healing Powers," *New York Times*, June 25, 2000, Women's Health, p. 6.

Samuels, Michael, M.D. *Healing with the Mind's Eye: A Guide for Using Imagery and Visions for Personal Growth and Healing*. New York: Summit Books, 1990.

Science and the Power of Prayer. 1999. Produced and directed by Elda Hartley. 55 min. Wellspring Media. Videocassette.

"Searching for Health Information Online." *Dr. Andrew Weil's Self Healing Newsletter*, January 2000: 2–3.

"Selenium: Anti-Cancer Buzz Brings Star Status to Once Maligned Mineral." *Environmental Nutrition* 22, no. 3 (March 1999).

Somerville, Robert, ed. *The Alternative Advisor: The Complete Guide to Natural and Alternative Treatments*. Alexandria, Va.: Time-Life Books, 1997.

"Sound Healing." *Dr. Andrew Weil's Self Healing Newsletter*, February 1998: 1, 6.

"Study Explores Health Benefits of Ancient Chinese Technique." *Inside the Institute: Dana-Farber Cancer Institute Newsletter*, January 11, 2000.

Szold, Henrietta. *Life of the Spirit*. New York: Atantia Productions, 1934.

Targ, Elisabeth, M.D. "Distant Healing." *IONS Noetic Science Review*, August–November 1999: 24–29.

"Ten Steps to Successful Surgery." *Dr. Andrew Weil's Self Healing Newsletter*, September 1997: 1, 6.

"Therapeutic Touch." *Dr. Andrew Weil's Self Healing Newsletter*, January 1998: 3.

Wager, Susan, M.D. *A Doctor's Guide to Therapeutic Touch*. New York: Perigee, 1996.

Yeager, Selene, and editors of Prevention Health Books, *New Foods for Healing*. Emmaus, Pa.: Rodale Press, Inc., 1998: 74–75, 106.

Zaharian, Beverly. *Activist Cancer Patient: How to Take Charge of Your Treatment*. New York: John Wiley and Sons, 1996.

Resources

In addition to resources listed within the text, you may contact the following organizations by phone, fax, or e-mail to learn more about specific topics or to locate a certified practitioner in your area.

Academy for Guided Imagery
(800) 726-2070
(415) 389-9324

ALCASE
(Alliance for Lung Cancer Advocacy,
Support, and Education)
(800) 298-2436
info@alcase.org

American Academy of Medical Acupuncture
(800) 521-2262
www.medicalacupuncture.org

American Council of Hypnotist Examiners
(818) 242-5378
(818) 247-9379 (fax)

American Holistic Nurse's Association
(800) 278-AHNA
www.ahna.org

American Massage Therapy Association
(847) 864-0123
www.amtamassage.org

American Polarity Therapy Association
(303) 545-2161

Ask Dr. Weil
www.drweil.com

Ask a Nurse
(800) 544-2424

Barbara Brennan School of Healing
(800) 924-2564
www.barbarabrennan.com

CancerSmart Newsletter
(800) 996-7522
(Memorial Sloan-Kettering Cancer Center)

Cancer Survivor Toolbox
Caring for the Caregiver Audiotape
(877) TOOLS-4U

Center for Human Caring
(303) 270-6157

Center for Journal Therapy
(888) 421-2298
www.journaltherapy.com

Commonweal Cancer Project
(415) 868-2642
(retreats)

Dialogue House Associates
(800) 221-5844
www.intensivejournal.org

Exceptional Cancer Patients Group
(814) 333-5060
www.ecap-online.org
(Dr. Bernie Siegel)

Friends Health Connection
(800) 48-FRIEND

Healing and Prayer Institute
(505) 820-5479
(Larry Dossey, M.D.)

Healing Touch International
(303) 989-7982
www.healingtouch.net

Insight Meditation Society
(508) 355-4378
(508) 355-6398 (fax)

Institute for Music, Health, and Education
(800) 490-4968
imhemn@pressenter.com

Institute of Noetic Sciences
(707) 775-3500

International Society for the Study of
Subtle Energies and Energy Medicine
74040.1273@compuserve.com

Jin Shin Iyutsu, Inc.
(602) 998-9331

Lauretta Laroche Videos
(508) 224-2280
(Humor Specialist, videos, and lectures)

Milton H. Erickson Foundation
(602) 956-6196
(602) 956-0519 (fax)
www.erickson.org

National Acupuncture and Oriental
Medicine Alliance
(253) 851-6896
www.acuall.org

National Cancer Coalition
(877) YES-NCCS
www.cansearch.org

National Certification Board for
Therapeutic Massage and Bodywork
(703) 610-9015

National Coalition for Cancer Survivorship
(301) 650-8868

Nurse Healers-Professional Associates International
(801) 273-3399
www.therapeutic-touch.org

Nutrition Hotline
(800) 843-8114

The Reiki Alliance
(208) 682-3535
(208) 682-4848 (fax)

Sound Healers Association
(303) 443-8181

Stress Reduction Tapes
www.mindfulnesstapes.com
(Jon Kabat-Zinn)

Survivorship Hotline
(877) 333-HOPE

Therapeutic Touch Nurse Healers Professional
Associates Cooperative
(412) 355-8476

Vipassana Meditation Center
(413) 625-2160

Wellspring Life Enhancement
(617) 929-0515
(visitation and training)

About the Author

MARGIE LEVINE is a health education teacher, social worker, and therapist who specializes in integrative medicine, which blends conventional and complementary therapies. She conducts mind/body seminars, as well as cancer workshops, and does personal counseling on health-related issues using her forty-one steps toward wellness. She also heads the Boston Institute of Noetic Science group, one of three hundred worldwide. Margie has presented her program to doctors at the Dana-Farber Cancer Institute, Brigham and Women's Hospital, and Newton-Wellesley Hospital, all in the Boston area. She divides her time between Boston and Cape Cod, Massachusetts.